Interventional Treatment for Structural Heart Disease

Edited by Takashi Murashita

Published in London, United Kingdom

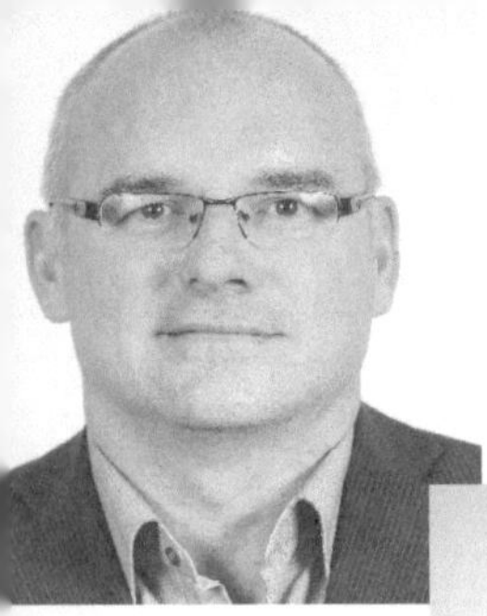
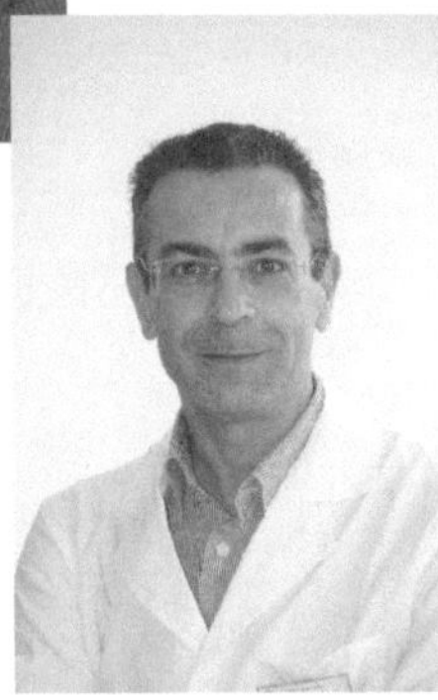
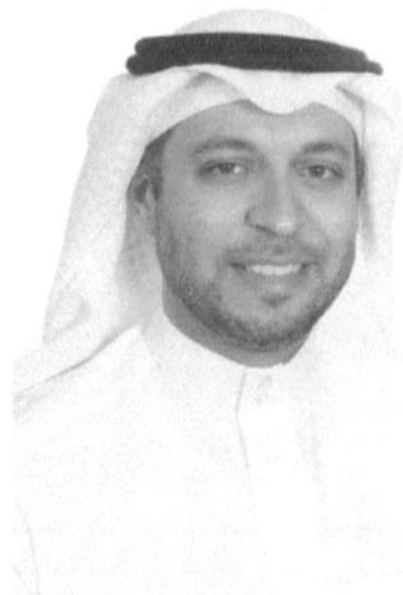
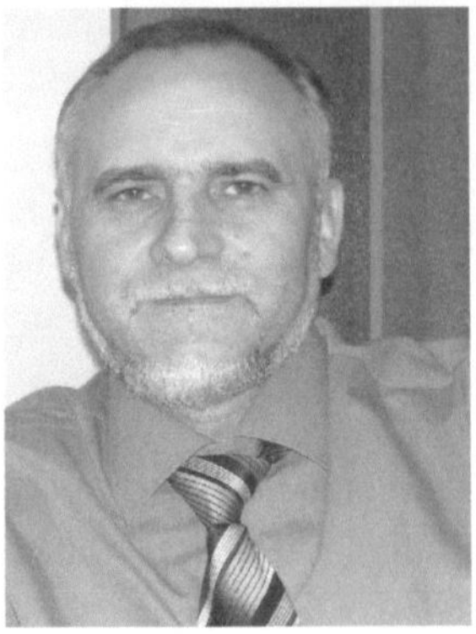
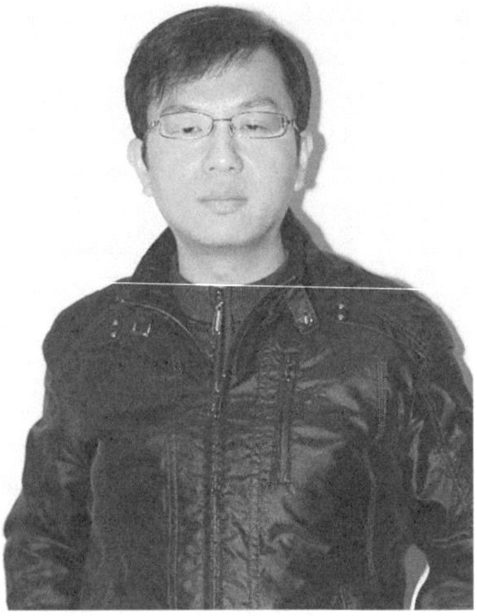
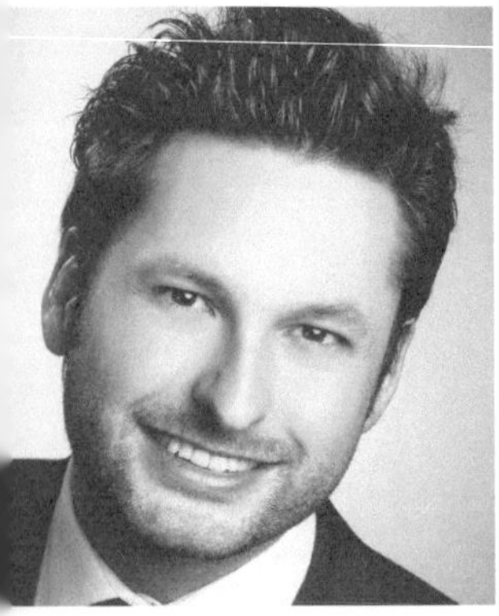
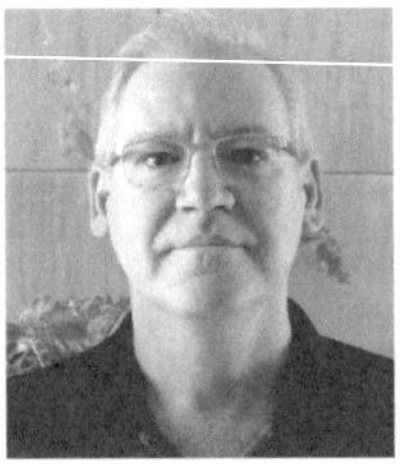

IntechOpen

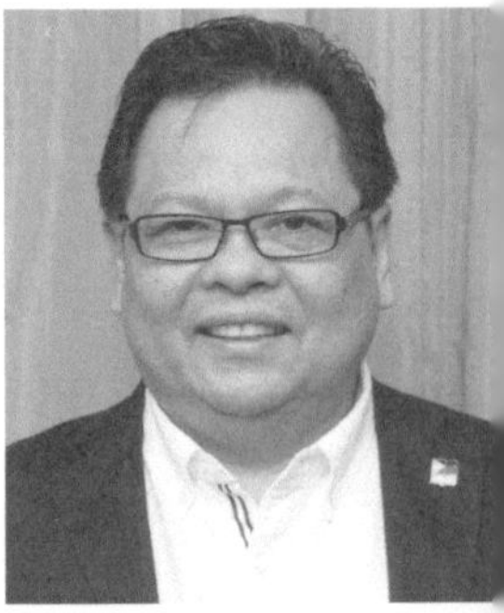
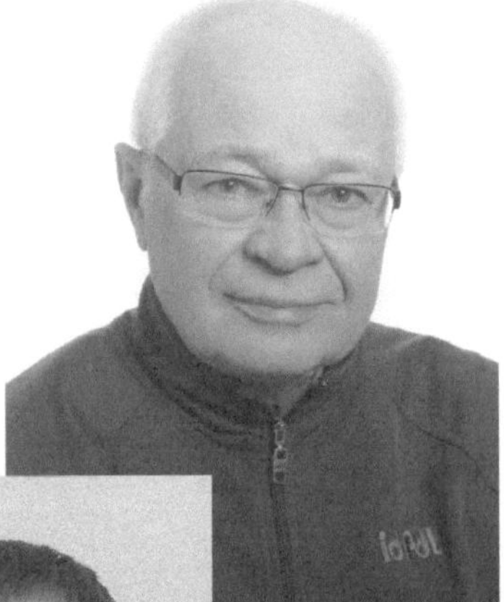
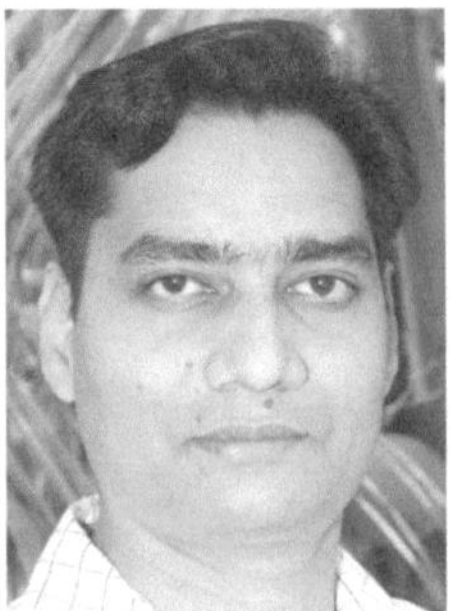
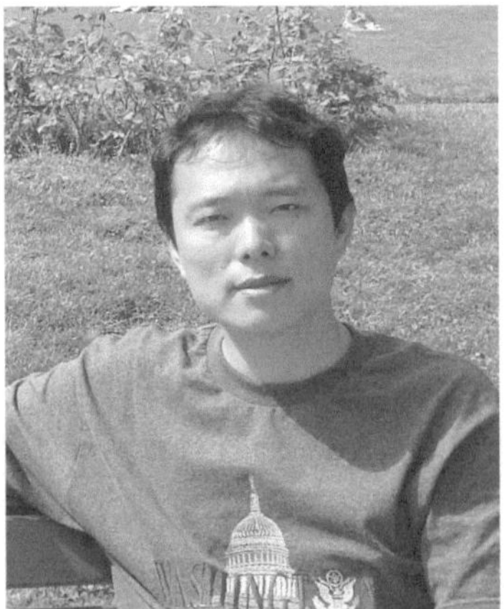
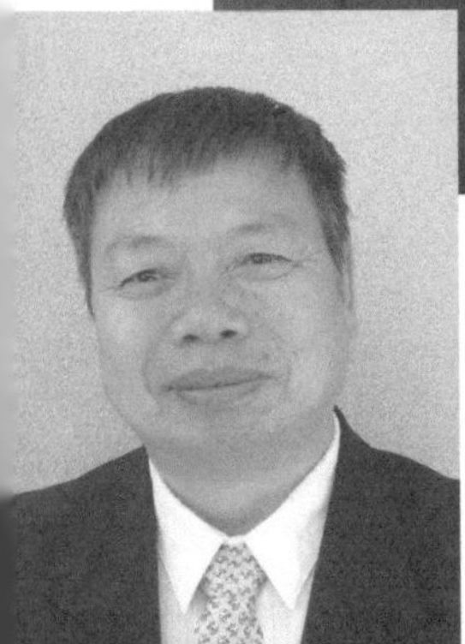
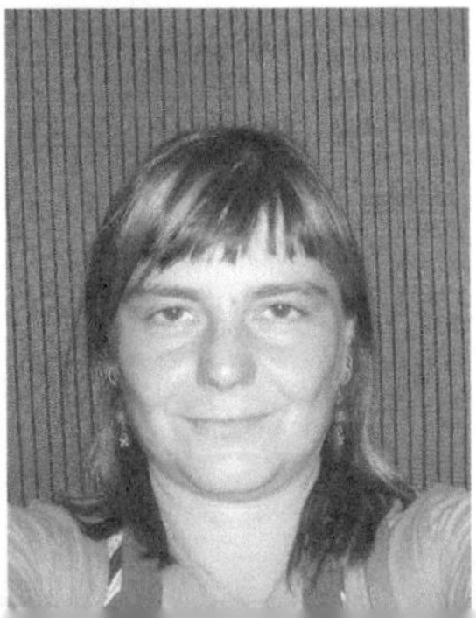

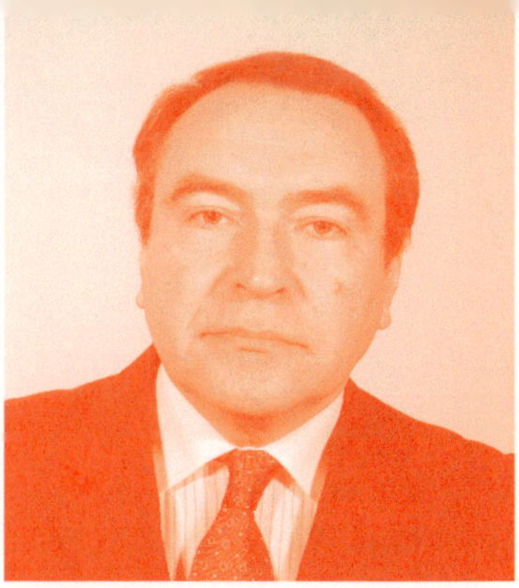
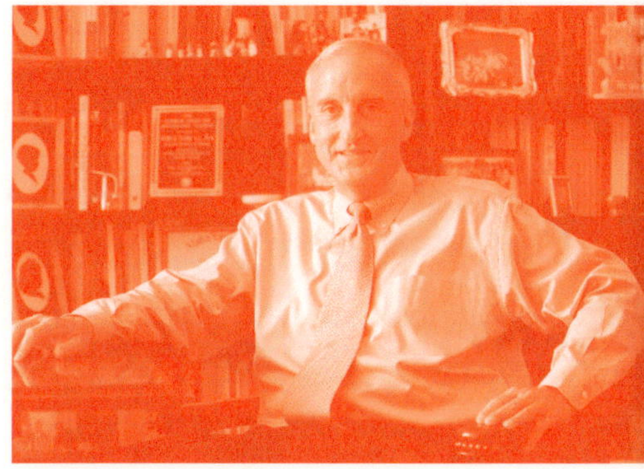
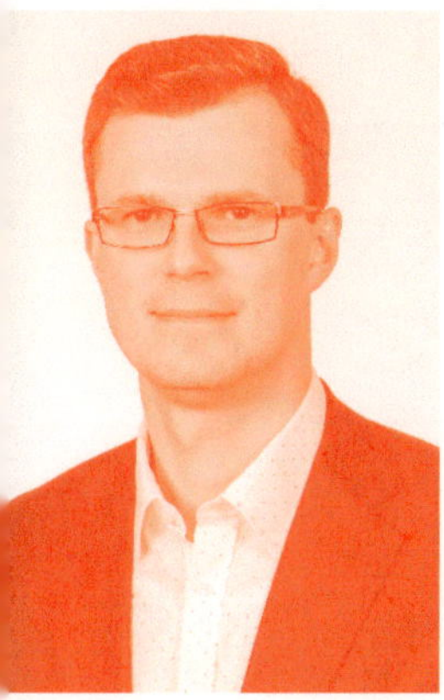
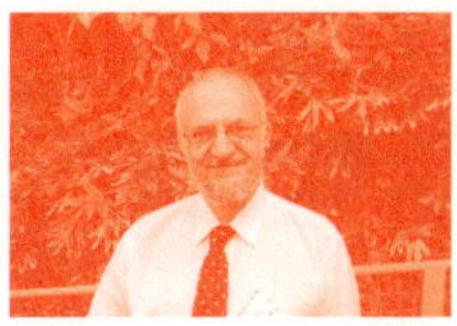
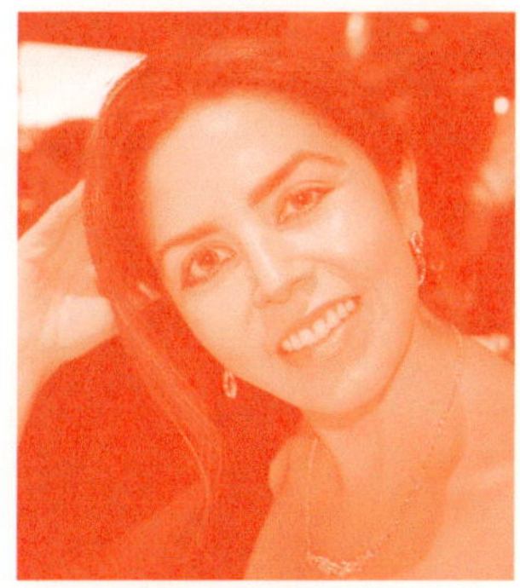

Supporting open minds since 2005

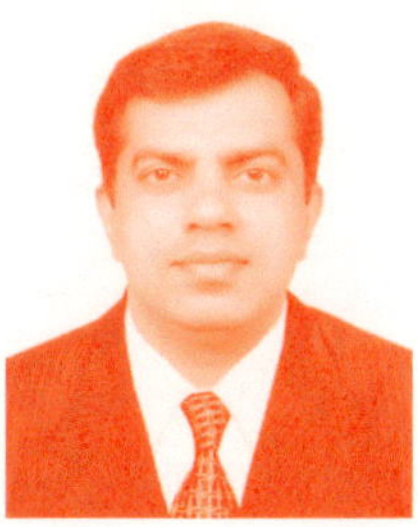
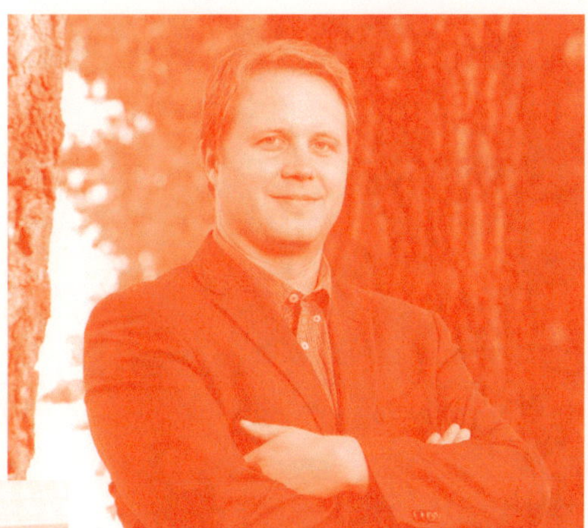
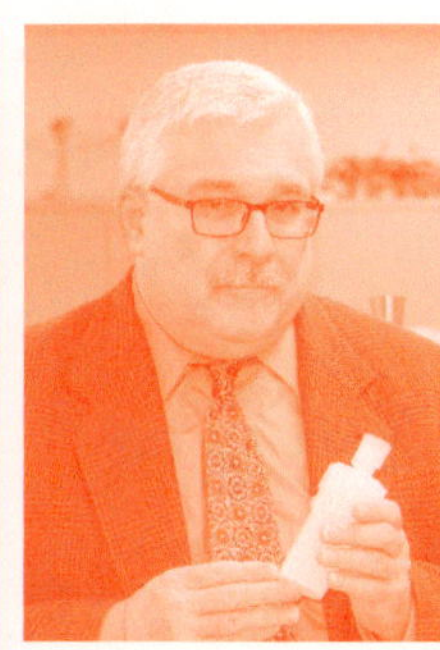
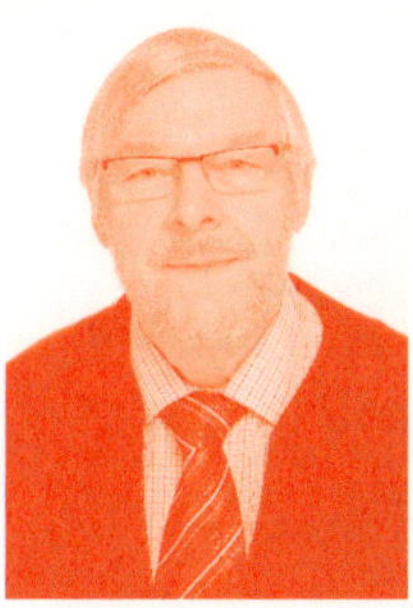
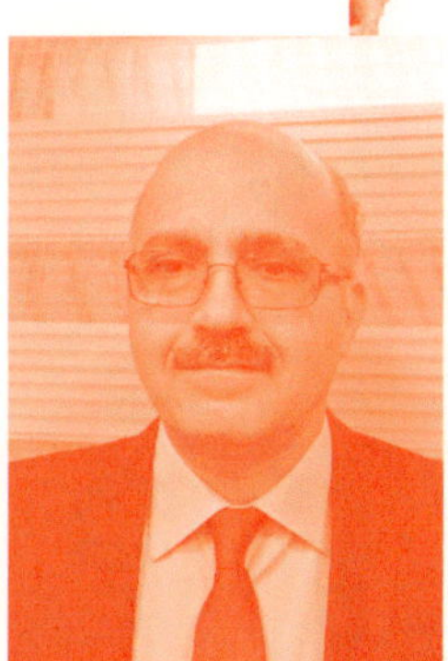
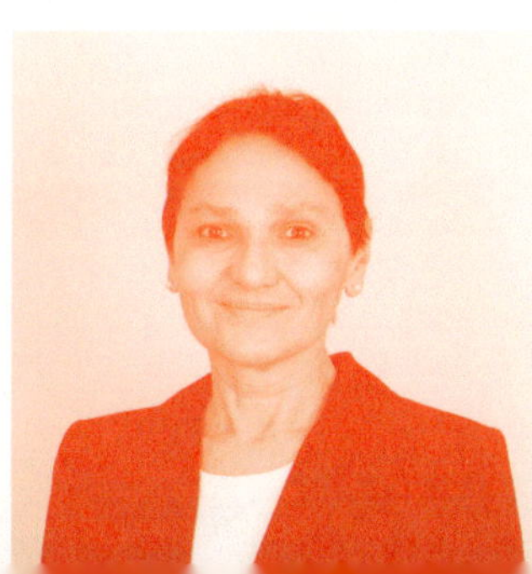
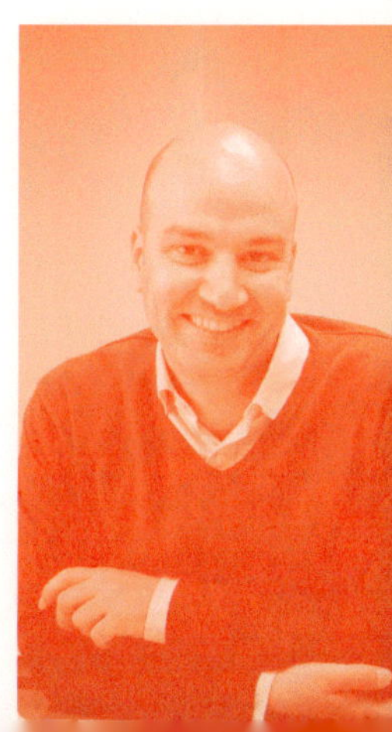

Interventional Treatment for Structural Heart Disease
http://dx.doi.org/10.5772/intechopen.91491
Edited by Takashi Murashita

Contributors
Tomás Benito-Gonzalez, Rodrigo Estévez-Loureiro, Felipe Fernández-Vázquez, Carmen Garrote-Coloma, Carlos Minguito-Carazo, Julio Echarte-Morales, Armando Pérez de Prado, Carmelo Panetta, Johnny Chahine, Jean-Francois Tanguay, Marcel Santaló-Corcoy, Guillaume Marquis-Gravel, Pilar Jimenez Quevedo, Carolina Espejo Paeres, Breda Hennessey, Manel Sabate, Takashi Murashita, Lina Ya'Qoub, Marvin Eng

First published in London, United Kingdom, 2021 by IntechOpen
IntechOpen is the global imprint of INTECHOPEN LIMITED, registered in England and Wales, registration number: 11086078, 5 Princes Gate Court, London, SW7 2QJ, United Kingdom
Printed in Croatia

British Library Cataloguing-in-Publication Data
A catalogue record for this book is available from the British Library

Additional hard and PDF copies can be obtained from orders@intechopen.com

Interventional Treatment for Structural Heart Disease
Edited by Takashi Murashita
p. cm.
Print ISBN 978-1-83968-363-3
Online ISBN 978-1-83968-364-0
eBook (PDF) ISBN 978-1-83968-365-7

Meet the editor

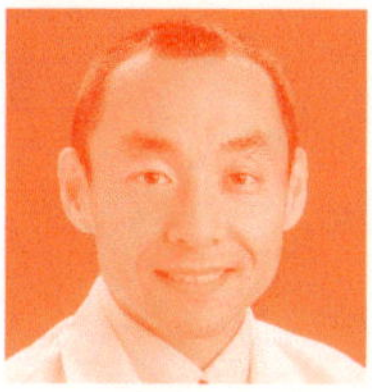

Takashi Murashita, MD, is an assistant professor in the Department of Surgery, University of Missouri, USA. Dr. Murashita received his MD from Kyoto University Medical School, Japan. His main interest is cardiac surgery, and he is a member of the Society of Thoracic Surgery, Eastern Cardiothoracic Surgical Society, and Asian Society for Cardiovascular and Thoracic Surgery. He has published fifty-three papers in peer-reviewed journals and ten book chapters. He has been an editorial board member and ad hoc manuscript reviewer for several medical journals.

Contents

Preface

Interventional Treatment for Structural Heart Disease is an excellent resource for healthcare professionals treating patients suffering from severe coronary artery disease and valvular disease. It includes six chapters over two sections.

The first section describes percutaneous coronary intervention for coronary artery disease. Chapter 1 presents recent research on dual antiplatelet therapy after percutaneous coronary intervention. The optimal duration of dual antiplatelet therapy is still controversial. Chapter 2 focuses on the outcome of percutaneous coronary intervention in patients with diabetes. Chapter 3 is a review of radial artery access at the time of coronary intervention.

The second section describes percutaneous valve replacement. Chapter 4 discusses the most recent updates in the field of valve-in-valve transcatheter aortic valve replacement. A significant trend toward the use of bioprostheses is leading to more patients with structural valve degeneration. Chapters 5 and 6 describe the most recent evidence in transcatheter mitral valve replacement and tricuspid valve replacement, respectively.

This book provides updated information about percutaneous intervention in coronary artery disease and valvular disease.

Takashi Murashita, MD
Assistant Professor,
Division of Cardiothoracic Surgery,
University of Missouri,
Columbia, MO, USA

Section 1

Percutaneous Coronary Intervention

Chapter 1

Dual Antiplatelet Therapy after PCI: When Could We Go Shorter?

Marcel Santaló-Corcoy, Guillaume Marquis-Gravel and Jean-François Tanguay

Abstract

The optimal duration of dual antiplatelet therapy (DAPT) after percutaneous coronary intervention (PCI) remains an important clinical question in interventional cardiology. Several clinical and angiographic variables are associated with an increased risk for thrombotic events, and prolonged DAPT duration may improve long term clinical outcome. However, some patients also present high bleeding risk (HBR) characteristics and may require a shorter DAPT duration. The guidelines recommendations consider the data from randomized clinical trials, however numerous exclusion criteria may create gaps in the evidence leading to uncertainties, the need for expert opinion and patient level decision making. Furthermore, the stent platforms have evolved in such way that opportunities now exist to shorten duration of DAPT. This chapter will review the variables associated with ischemic and bleeding risks as well as different stent platforms to help clinicians optimize DAPT duration in patients undergoing PCI.

Keywords: percutaneous coronary intervention, stents, acute coronary syndrome, high bleeding risk, duration of antiplatelet therapy

1. Introduction

The optimal antiplatelet therapy after percutaneous coronary intervention (PCI) remains an unanswered clinical question. The last 25 years of clinical investigations has mainly been focused on the choice of P2Y12 agents and on treatment duration. Initially, the observation that bare metal stents (BMS) implantation could be associated with thrombosis, and, subsequently, the observation that first-generation drug eluting stents (DES) were associated with very-late thrombosis risk led to studies evaluating prolonged duration regimens of DAPT after PCI, but also to innovations in stent technology. However, the newer, more potent drugs (prasugrel and ticagrelor) and the advent and evolution of modern second- and third-generation DES dramatically dwindled the incidence of late and very late thrombotic complications. Thus, interest has shifted in trying to find the optimal, shortened DAPT treatment to prevent the early thrombotic complications while avoiding the late hemorrhagic events, the latter being associated with a similar risk of all-cause mortality than post-PCI recurrent myocardial infarctions [1].

Numerous trials attempted to answer these important questions, sometimes leading to discrepant results. This chapter will focus on the current evidence listed on the guidelines of main scientific societies for three groups of patients: elective PCI,

PCI in the setting of acute coronary syndromes (ACS), and PCI for patients with a coexisting indication of oral anticoagulation (OAC). For each of them we will highlight the standard recommendations for DAPT duration, as well as the main clinical, angiographic and stent-derived variables that should be used in the decision-making process to tailor a shortened DAPT therapy reflecting each patient need.

2. Latest guidelines on the topic

This document will include the latest recommendations of Canadian, American and European guidelines. Canadian scientific societies published two documents in 2018 addressing antithrombotic treatment: The Canadian Cardiovascular Society (CCS)/Canadian Association of Interventional Cardiology focused update for the use of antiplatelet therapy [2] and the CCS focused update for the management of atrial fibrillation [3]. The American College of Cardiology/American Heart Association (ACC/AHA) published a focused update on the duration of DAPT in patients with coronary artery disease (CAD) in 2016, [4] while a recent AHA/ACC/Heart Rhythm Society (HRS) focused update in the management of patients with atrial fibrillation was published in 2019 [5]. Lastly, the European Society of Cardiology (ESC) and European Association for Cardio-Thoracic Surgery (EACTS) published a focused update on DAPT in 2017 [6]. However, the most recent 2020 ESC guidelines for management of ACS in patients presenting without persistent ST-segment elevation [7] and 2020 ESC/EACTS guidelines for the management of atrial fibrillation [8] will also be reviewed. A dedicated, critical comparison of the available guidelines on DAPT was published previously this year [9].

3. Evaluation of bleeding and thrombotic risk

In order to tailor optimal DAPT duration, many variables must be taken into account to ensure adequate thrombotic protection while avoiding hemorrhagic complications. To that extent, different risk scores have been derived and validated.

The PARIS risk score was one of the first tools intended to predict risks for out-of-hospital events directly modified by prolonging DAPT beyond one year (i.e. coronary thrombosis and bleeding) [10]. The aim of the DAPT score is to identify patients expected to derive benefit or harm from continuing $P2Y_{12}$ beyond 1 year. To that extent, data was gathered among patients that had not experienced any major ischemic or bleeding event 12 months after the index procedure [11]. Similarly, the CALIBER score includes patients surviving 12 months after a MI, including those not treated with PCI [12]. Hence, these three risk scores help establishing the security of long term DAPT duration.

In contrast, the PRECISE-DAPT score [13] assesses the benefit of a short (3–6 month) versus a long (12–24 month) DAPT duration. Furthermore, it allows clinicians to select DAPT duration upfront instead of at another point in time during follow-up. Of note, patients with the need of OAC were excluded from the derivation cohort. Patients undergoing elective, urgent and emergent PCI were all included in the analysis. At the time of the index PCI, an additive score is calculated by means of the presence of five clinical and biochemical variables (age, creatinine clearance, hemoglobin, white blood cell count and prior spontaneous bleeding), ranging 0 to 100 points. Patients $\geq$25 points were considered high bleeding risk (HBR), while <25 points were defined as non-HBR. Among HBR patients based on this score, prolonged DAPT contributed to no significant ischemic benefit, while, on the other hand, led to an increased risk of bleeding (number to harm

(NNH) = 38). In parallel, non-HBR patients benefited of a longer DAPT regimen in the form of a significant reduction in the composite endpoint of myocardial infarction (MI), definite stent thrombosis, stroke and target vessel revascularization (NNT for benefit of 68), with no significant increase in bleeding risk [13]. Results were consistent across the full spectrum of indications for PCI.

Some works have compared the accuracy of these scores head-to-head, in general showing little to no difference in their ability to predict bleeding [14–16].

More recently, the new ARC-HBR criteria have been validated at identifying patients at high bleeding risk, being more sensitive than the PRECISE-DAPT and PARIS risk scores (at the expense of specificity) [17]. Trials where these criteria are used to compare different antiplatelet durations are awaited.

It is worth noting, however, that no prediction model has been prospectively tested in the setting of a RCT.

On the other side of the coin, clinicians should be aware of certain clinical and angiographic features associated with a higher thrombotic risk in some patients, thus making it unadvisable to shorten their antiplatelet regimens. These characteristics are summarized in **Table 2**.

4. Evidence for DAPT duration after PCI in non-ACS setting

Many trials have demonstrated the non-inferiority of 6-month versus longer treatment duration amid "all-comer" patients undergoing PCI for stable and ACS settings, [18–22] and so the recommendations for elective PCI are extrapolated for the aggregated results. The ACC and ESC guidelines give strong recommendations on a standard 6-month duration of DAPT in stable patients. As for the CCS, it places greater emphasis on reduction of major CV thrombotic events vs. an increase in bleeding complications, by recommending DAPT duration from 6 up to 12 months. (**Table 1**) This is due to some metanalysis showing increased risk of ischemic outcomes with shorter DAPT durations in certain groups with high risk angiographic features (**Table 2**) [24–26].

All three guidelines suggest considering a 3-month DAPT course in patients at HBR. This comes from the experience of two trials where a zotarolimus-eluting stent was tested [27, 28]. However, due to the fact that this platform is no longer available, the recommendation stands at a weak level of evidence. The ESC guidelines also include the possibility of a 1-month period of DAPT in patients in whom 3-month DAPT poses safety concerns. This recommendation comes from two trials in which a zotarolimus-eluting Endeavor sprint stent or Biofreedom drug-coated stent reduced ischemic endpoints compared to bare-metal stent under similar DAPT duration [29, 30].

Since their publication, some new evidence supports aspirin-free strategies early after PCI: the TWILIGHT trial included high risk patients who had not had an ischemic or bleeding event after a three-month course of aspirin plus ticagrelor and randomized them to aspirin or placebo for one year. Patients with ticagrelor monotherapy had a lower clinically relevant bleeding incidence while providing no higher death or ischemic endpoints [31]. The SMART-CHOICE randomized patients to receive aspirin plus a P2Y12 inhibitor for 3 months and thereafter a P2Y12 inhibitor alone or DAPT por 12 months. The monotherapy arm resulted in noninferior rates of major adverse cardiac events [32].

The GLOBAL LEADERS trial assessed the combination of ticagrelor and aspirin for one month followed by ticagrelor alone for 23 month versus 12 months of standard DAPT followed by 12 month of aspirin alone, with neutral results [33]. Later, its ancillary substudy (GLASSY) showed the non-inferiority, but not superiority,

		DAPT duration	Grade of recommendation	DAPT duration	Grade of recommendation	DAPT duration	Grade of recommendation
		CCS – 2017 [3]		**ACC/AHA – 2016** [4]		**ESC – 2017** [6]	
DES-PCI for stable patients	Standard duration	6–12 months	Strong recommendation, moderate-quality evidence	6 months	Class I, level B-R	6 months	Class I, level A
	Minimal duration	3 months (HBR)	Weak recommendation, low-quality evidence	3 months (HBR or overt bleeding)	Class IIb, level C-LD	3 months (HBR)	Class IIa, level B
						1 month (if bleeding safety concern with 3-month DAPT)	Class IIb, level C
		CCS – 2017 [3]		**ACC/AHA – 2016** [4]		**ESC – 2020** [7]	
DES-PCI for ACS	Standard duration	12 months	Strong recommendation, high-quality evidence	12 months	Class I, level B-R	12 months	Class I, level A
	Minimal duration	12 months	Strong recommendation, high-quality evidence	6 months	Class IIb, level C-LD	3 months (HBR)	Class IIa, level B
						3–6 months, depending on ischemic/bleeding risk balance	Class IIa, level A

Table 1.
Standard and shortened DAPT duration according to different guidelines. Adapted and updated from [9].

Clinical [23]
Previous myocardial infarction
Diabetes mellitus
Chronic kidney disease (creatinine clearance <60 mL/min)
Previous stent thrombosis
Current smoker
Angiographic
Implantation of ≥3 stents [24]
Stented length (>60 mm) [24]
Complex lesions (bifurcation, chronic total occlusion) [24]
Left main or left anterior descending stenting [25]
Multivessel stenting [26]

Table 2.
High risk features associated with thrombotic events. Adapted from [3].

of shortened DAPT arm in a selected subpopulation of the 20 highest recruiting sites of the main trial [34]. On the other hand, the STOPDAPT-2 trial showed the benefit of 1 month of aspirin plus clopidogrel followed by clopidogrel monotherapy vs. 12 month of standard DAPT, meeting the criteria for both noninferiority and superiority [35].

5. Evidence for DAPT duration after PCI in ACS setting

The three sets of guidelines provide strong recommendation for a standard 12-month DAPT treatment after an ACS, based on the CURE trial and the PCI-CURE substudy published nearly two decades ago, in which DAPT with aspirin and clopidogrel was prescribed for 3 to 12 months after PCI [36, 37]. More recently, the pivotal prasugrel and ticagrelor trials, conducted in patients with ACS, used a 12-month default DAPT duration, furthermore establishing this approach as the standard of practice (**Table 1**) [38, 39].

5.1 Scenarios for shortened DAPT

Due to the time gap between the latest ESC guidelines on this topic and its American and Canadian counterparts, recommendations on minimal DAPT duration differ between the former and the latter (**Table 1**). The scarce evidence available at the time of the last ACC/AHA and CCS guidelines led to only weak recommendation for a 6-month DAPT on the former, while the latter holds at a 12-month recommendation. This year's ESC guidelines on the management of ACS in patients presenting without persisting ST-segment elevation includes various guidance on short DAPT.

As discussed previously, the insight from the PRECISE-DAPT study led to consider a shortened 3-month DAPT duration in patients at HBR (PRECISE-DAPT score ≥ 25) (Recommendation IIa B) [13]. What is probably more interesting, however, is the evidence gathered recently on patients at low-to-intermediate ischemic risk and low bleeding risk. The previously described TWILIGHT and SMART-CHOICE trials included a high proportion of patients presenting with ACS (64.8% and 58.2%, respectively), with the benefits of antiplatelet monotherapy being consistent between subgroups. On the other hand, the SMART-DATE trial [40] specifically assessed 6 versus 12-month DAPT in patients with ACS. Although mortality, stroke and BARC type 2–5 bleeding did not differ between the two groups, the rate of myocardial infarction was higher in the short DAPT group. Combining the information of these three trials, the ESC guidelines suggest a 3 to 6-month DAPT therapy depending on the balance of ischemic and hemorrhagic risk in a Class IIa, level A recommendation. The recent TICO trial evaluated another aspirin-free strategy, specifically among patients undergoing PCI for an ACS [41]. Ticagrelor monotherapy after 3 months of DAPT resulted in a slight, significant reduction of the composite outcome of major bleeding and cardiovascular events at one year, compared with a ticagrelor-based 12-month DAPT.

6. Evidence of shortened DAPT duration in patients after PCI requiring lifelong oral anticoagulation

The landscape of evidence for the treatment of patients requiring lifelong oral anticoagulation after PCI has expanded notably in the last years, the main landmarks being (1) the ISAR-TRIPLE trial, where no significant difference was found in the primary endpoint of "net clinical benefit" (which included ischemic and bleeding outcomes) between 6 weeks and six months of triple therapy; [42] (2) the WOEST trial, where a dual pathway strategy (warfarin and clopidogrel) versus standard triple therapy (warfarin, clopidogrel and ASA) reduced bleeding while not increasing thrombotic events; [43] and (3) the advent of the new four direct oral anticoagulants (DOAC) and their specific trials for patients undergoing PCI,

AF patients with ACS/PCI		
Clinical setting	**Therapy regimen**	**Recommendation**
Uncomplicated or bleeding[a] > ischemic[b] risk	• TT < 1 week • OAC + P2Y12 (preferably clopidogrel) up to 12 months	I B
Ischemic[b] > bleeding[a] risk	• TT > 1 week and ≤ 1 month • OAC + P2Y12 (preferably clopidogrel) up to 12 months	IIa C
AF patients with CCS undergoing PCI		
Clinical setting	**Therapy regimen**	**Recommendation**
Uncomplicated or bleeding[a] > ischemic[b] risk	• TT ≤ 1 week • OAC + P2Y12 (preferably clopidogrel) up to 6 months	I B
Ischemic[b] > bleeding[a] risk	• TT > 1 week and ≤ 1 month • OAC + clopidogrel up to 12 months	IIa C

[a]*Evaluation based on HAS-BLED score: Hypertension, Abnormal renal or liver function, Stroke or ICH history, Bleeding history or bleeding diathesis, Labile INR, Elderly (>65 years), Drugs (concomitant OAC and antiplatelet therapy, NSAIDs).*
[b]*Evaluation based on (1) clinical factors: diabetes, prior ACS, multivessel CAD, concomitant peripheral artery disease, premature or accelerated CAD, chronic kidney disease, ACS as clinical presentation; (2) anatomical factors: multivessel stenting, complex stenting (left main or last patent vessel stenting, chronic total occlusion intervention), prior stent thrombosis on antiplatelet treatment.*
TT: Triple therapy; CCS: chronic coronary syndrome.

Table 3.
Recommendations for antithrombotic patients of AF patients undergoing PCI. Adapted from the 2020 ESC ESC/EACTS guidelines for the management of atrial fibrillation [8].

[dabigatran/RE-DUAL PCI [44]; rivaroxaban/PIONEER AF-PCI [45]; apixaban/AUGUSTUS [46]; edoxaban/ENTRUST-AF PCI [47]. The new 2020 ESC ESC/EACTS guidelines for the management of atrial fibrillation is the latest consensus document on the subject, and the only one after the publication of the four DOAC trials for AF patients undergoing PCI [8].

As a whole, these trials evaluated dual (DOAC + $P2Y_{12}$) vs. triple (VKA + $P2Y_{12}$ + aspirin) therapy. They included a notable proportion of ACS (37–52%), although the highest risk patients were underrepresented (i.e., culprit lesions in a previously stented segment). Moreover, they all used triple therapy during PCI until randomization (1–14 days post PCI) and the most commonly $P2Y_{12}$ inhibitor used was clopidogrel, as neither prasugrel or ticagrelor have evidence supporting their safety in combination with an OAC. As per outcomes, they reported a significant reduction of major/clinically significant bleeding, comparable rates of ischemic stroke, similar or non-significantly higher rates of myocardial infarction and stent thrombosis and a neutral effect on major adverse cardiac events and all-cause mortality [48]. Also, it is worth emphasizing that the AUGUSTUS trial is the only one that studied whether the advantages of dual pathway (vs. triple therapy) is independent of the type of OAC.

The ESC guidelines include four recommendations, according to the clinical presentation and the ischemic/bleeding risk balance (**Table 3**). Due to the under-representation of high ischemic risk patients on the trials, the recommendations for this population have a weak level of evidence. The evaluation of the ischemic risk is based on the presence of variables known to pose higher risk in the general population (also previously described in **Table 2**). Regarding the bleeding risk, evaluation with the AF-specific HAS-BLED risk score is recommended. This bleeding risk score has proven to be more useful at predicting bleeding risk in AF patients [49].

7. Beyond guidelines: tailored shortened DAPT durations according to stent platforms

Current guidelines include DAPT length recommendations irrespective of the DES type, encompassing the evidence of the multiple platforms in various trials. It is worth mentioning, however, some recent trials in which specific platforms have been tested in two main scenarios: one stent tested at short vs. longer DAPT durations; and two different stents compared in a short DAPT duration for patients not deemed amenable for prolonged DAPT duration. While acknowledging the limited value of a single trial, they may still be useful for tailored antiplatelet regimens. **Table 4** summarizes the current knowledge of some specific DES platforms in these two scenarios.

8. Conclusions

As new antiplatelet and anticoagulant drugs have entered the therapeutic arsenal, and as stent platforms continue to be refined through the years, established dogmas of the treatment of patients with ischemic heart disease should be reassessed. Most notably, current evidence strongly supports that for a considerable number of patients, shorter antithrombotic, aspirin-free treatment is associated not only with fewer bleeding complications, but with comparable rates of hard ischemic endpoints. Hence, a paradigm shift is underway, in which the concern should not be to find reasons to reduce the classical 12 months of DAPT. Rather, patients should be evaluated for causes *not to* receive an abbreviated aspirin-free antithrombotic

Trial	Stent platform	Population study	Study arms and DAPT therapy	Outcomes
Trials testing short vs. long DAPT durations in patients treated with new stent platforms				
GLOBAL LEADERS [33]	BioMatrix (Biosensors Europe)	All comers	Biomatrix stent 1 month DAPT ASA + ticagrelor followed by ticagrelor 12 months vs. DAPT ASA + clopidogrel (stable patients) or ASA/ ticagrelor (ACS) followed by ASA (1:1)	No superiority of the ticagrelor arm for efficacy
COBRA-REDUCE [50]	Cobra PzF (CeloNova Biosciences)	Patients taking OAC	Cobra stent vs. standard DES Cobra: DAPT 14 days, then OAC + ASA until 6 monts. Control stent: DAPT 3–6 monts. After 6 months, all received OAC + ASA	Cobra PzF stents did not achieve bleeding reduction and did not meet non-inferiority criteria with respect to thrombotic events
XIENCE 90/28 [51]	Xience (Abbott Vascular)	High bleeding risk	Xience stent DAPT 1 month and DAPT 3 months, compared to historical cohort DAPT 12 months	Non-inferior ischemic outcomes, similar rates of clinically relevant and reduction in major bleeding
EVOLVE Short DAPT [52]	Synergy (Boston Scientific)	High bleeding risk	Synergy stent 3 month DAPT vs. 12 month historical cohort	Non inferior ischemic outcomes
TICO [41]	Orsiro (Biotronik AG)	Acute coronary syndromes	Orsiro stent 3 month DAPT followed by ticagrelor monotherapy vs standard 12 month DAPT	Modest reduction of bleeding and cardiovascular events.
Trials testing different stent technologies in patients deemed for short DAPT				
LEADERS FREE [30]	Biofreedom (Biosensors Europe)	High bleeding risk	Biofreedom vs. similar BMS (1:1) 1 month DAPT ASA + clopidogrel followed by clopidogrel	Superiority of the Biofreedom stent in safety and efficacy
ONYX ONE [53]	Resolute Onyx (Medtronic)	High bleeding risk	Resolute Onyx vs. Biofreedom (1:1) 1 month DAPT followed by SAPT	Resolute Onyx non-inferior to Biofreedom in safety and effectiveness
ZEUS [29]	Endeavor (Medtronic)	High bleeding risk	Endeavor stent vs. ultra-thin BMS (1:1) 1 month DAPT	Low risk of 1-year MACE in Endeavor patients
SENIOR [54]	Synergy (Boston Scientific)	Elderly patients (>75 yo) undergoing PCI	Synergy stent vs. ultrathin BMS 1 month or 6 months DAPT, according to stable or unstable presentation	Low risk of ischemic endpoints in the Synergy arm

Table 4.
Recent trials on the performance of different stent platforms on shortened DAPT scenarios.

regimen. In order to provide the most accurate treatment regimens, a careful evaluation should be made by taking into account the clinical presentation, coexisting conditions that are prone to a higher ischemic or bleeding risk and awareness of the stent platform used.

Author details

Marcel Santaló-Corcoy, Guillaume Marquis-Gravel and Jean-François Tanguay*
Montreal Heart Institute, Université de Montréal, Montréal, Canada

*Address all correspondence to: jean-francois.tanguay@icm-mhi.org

References

[1] Marquis-Gravel G, Dalgaard F, Jones AD, et al. Post-Discharge Bleeding and Mortality Following Acute Coronary Syndromes With or Without PCI. J. Am. Coll. Cardiol. 2020;76:162-171.

[2] Mehta SR, Bainey KR, Cantor WJ, et al. 2018 Canadian Cardiovascular Society/Canadian Association of Interventional Cardiology Focused Update of the Guidelines for the Use of Antiplatelet Therapy. Can. J. Cardiol. 2018;34:214-233.

[3] Andrade JG, Verma A, Mitchell LB, et al. 2018 Focused Update of the Canadian Cardiovascular Society Guidelines for the Management of Atrial Fibrillation. Can. J. Cardiol. 2018;34:1371-1392.

[4] Levine GN, Bates ER, Bittl JA, et al. 2016 ACC/AHA guideline focused update on duration of dual antiplatelet therapy in patients with coronary artery disease. J. Thorac. Cardiovasc. Surg. 2016;152:1243-1275.

[5] January CT, Wann LS, Calkins H, et al. 2019 AHA/ACC/HRS focused update of the 2014 AHA/ACC/HRS guideline for the management of patients with atrial fibrillation. Hear. Rhythm 2019;16:e66–e93.

[6] Valgimigli M, Bueno H, Byrne RA, et al. 2017 ESC focused update on dual antiplatelet therapy in coronary artery disease developed in collaboration with EACTS. Eur. J. Cardio-thoracic Surg. 2018;53:34-78.

[7] Collet J-P, Thiele H, Barbato E, et al. 2020 ESC Guidelines for the management of acute coronary syndromes in patients presenting without persistent ST-segment elevation. Eur. Heart J. 2020:1-79.

[8] Hindricks G, Potpara T, Dagres N, et al. 2020 ESC Guidelines for the diagnosis and management of atrial fibrillation developed in collaboration with the European Association of Cardio-Thoracic Surgery (EACTS). Eur. Heart J. 2020:1-126.

[9] Marquis-Gravel G, Mehta SR, Valgimigli M, et al. A Critical Comparison of Canadian and International Guidelines Recommendations for Antiplatelet Therapy in Coronary Artery Disease. Can. J. Cardiol. 2020;36:1298-1307. Available at: http://www.ncbi.nlm.nih.gov/pubmed/32553812.

[10] Baber U, Mehran R, Giustino G, et al. Coronary Thrombosis and Major Bleeding after PCI with Drug-Eluting Stents Risk Scores from Paris. J. Am. Coll. Cardiol. 2016;67:2224-2234.

[11] Yeh RW, Secemsky EA, Kereiakes DJ, et al. Development and validation of a prediction rule for benefit and harm of Dual antiplatelet therapy beyond 1 year after percutaneous coronary intervention. JAMA - J. Am. Med. Assoc. 2016;315:1735-1749.

[12] Pasea L, Chung SC, Pujades-Rodriguez M, et al. Personalising the decision for prolonged dual antiplatelet therapy: Development, validation and potential impact of prognostic models for cardiovascular events and bleeding in myocardial infarction survivors. Eur. Heart J. 2017;38:1048-1055.

[13] Costa F, van Klaveren D, James S, et al. Derivation and validation of the predicting bleeding complications in patients undergoing stent implantation and subsequent dual antiplatelet therapy (PRECISE-DAPT) score: a pooled analysis of individual-patient datasets from clinical trials. Lancet 2017;389:1025-1034.

[14] Bianco M, D'ascenzo F, Raposeiras Roubin S, et al. Comparative external validation of the PRECISE-DAPT and PARIS risk scores in 4424 acute

coronary syndrome patients treated with prasugrel or ticagrelor. Int. J. Cardiol. 2020;301:200-206. Available at: https://linkinghub.elsevier.com/retrieve/pii/S0167527319309891.

[15] Marquis-Gravel G, Neely ML, Valgimigli M, et al. Long-Term Bleeding Risk Prediction with Dual Antiplatelet Therapy after Acute Coronary Syndromes Treated without Revascularization. Circ. Cardiovasc. Qual. Outcomes 2020:627-638.

[16] Abu-Assi E, Raposeiras-Roubin S, Cobas-Paz R, et al. Assessing the performance of the PRECISE-DAPT and Paris risk scores for predicting one-year out-of-hospital bleeding in acute coronary syndrome patients. EuroIntervention 2018;13:1914-1922.

[17] Ueki Y, Bär S, Losdat S, et al. Validation of the Academic Research Consortium for High Bleeding Risk (ARC-HBR) criteria in patients undergoing percutaneous coronary intervention and comparison with contemporary bleeding risk scores. EuroIntervention 2020;16:371-379.

[18] Bertrand ME, Legrand V, Boland J, et al. Randomized multicenter comparison of conventional anticoagulation versus antiplatelet therapy in unplanned and elective coronary stenting. The full anticoagulation versus aspirin and ticlopidine (FANTASTIC) study. Circulation 1998;98:1597-1603.

[19] Colombo A, Chieffo A, Frasheri A, et al. Second-generation drug-eluting stent implantation followed by 6- versus 12-month dual antiplatelet therapy: the SECURITY randomized clinical trial. J. Am. Coll. Cardiol. 64:2086-97. Available at: http://www.ncbi.nlm.nih.gov/pubmed/25236346.

[20] Gwon H-C, Hahn J-Y, Park KW, et al. Six-month versus 12-month dual antiplatelet therapy after implantation of drug-eluting stents: the Efficacy of Xience/Promus Versus Cypher to Reduce Late Loss After Stenting (EXCELLENT) randomized, multicenter study. Circulation 2012;125:505-13. Available at: http://www.ncbi.nlm.nih.gov/pubmed/22179532.

[21] Schulz-Schüpke S, Byrne RA, Ten Berg JM, et al. ISAR-SAFE: A randomized, double-blind, placebo-controlled trial of 6 vs. 12 months of clopidogrel therapy after drug-eluting stenting. Eur. Heart J. 2015;36:1252-1263.

[22] Valgimigli M, Campo G, Monti M, et al. Short-versus long-term duration of dual-antiplatelet therapy after coronary stenting: A randomized multicenter trial. Circulation 2012;125:2015-2026.

[23] Bonaca MP, Bhatt DL, Cohen M, et al. Long-Term Use of Ticagrelor in Patients with Prior Myocardial Infarction. N. Engl. J. Med. 2015;372:1791-1800.

[24] Giustino G, Chieffo A, Palmerini T, et al. Efficacy and Safety of Dual Antiplatelet Therapy After Complex PCI. J. Am. Coll. Cardiol. 2016;68: 1851-1864.

[25] Costa F, Adamo M, Ariotti S, et al. Left main or proximal left anterior descending coronary artery disease location identifies high-risk patients deriving potentially greater benefit from prolonged dual antiplatelet therapy duration. EuroIntervention 2016;11:e1222–e1230.

[26] Lee SY, Hong MK, Shin DH, et al. Association between Duration of Dual Antiplatelet Therapy and Angiographic Multivessel Disease on Outcomes in Patients Treated with Newer-Generation Drug-Eluting Stents. Circ. Cardiovasc. Interv. 2016;9.

[27] Kim B-K, Hong M-K, Shin D-H, et al. A New Strategy for Discontinuation of Dual Antiplatelet Therapy. J. Am. Coll. Cardiol. 2012;60:1340-1348.

[28] Feres F, Costa RA, Abizaid A, et al. Three vs twelve months of dual antiplatelet therapy after zotarolimus-eluting stents: The OPTIMIZE randomized trial. JAMA - J. Am. Med. Assoc. 2013;310:2510-2522.

[29] Valgimigli M, Patialiakas A, Thury A, et al. Zotarolimus-eluting versus bare-metal stents in uncertain drug-eluting stent candidates. J. Am. Coll. Cardiol. 2015;65:805-815.

[30] Urban P, Meredith IT, Abizaid A, et al. Polymer-free Drug-Coated Coronary Stents in Patients at High Bleeding Risk. N. Engl. J. Med. 2015;373:2038-2047.

[31] Mehran R, Baber U, Sharma SK, et al. Ticagrelor with or without aspirin in high-risk patients after PCI. N. Engl. J. Med. 2019;381:2032-2042.

[32] Hahn JY, Song Y Bin, Oh JH, et al. Effect of P2Y12 Inhibitor Monotherapy vs Dual Antiplatelet Therapy on Cardiovascular Events in Patients Undergoing Percutaneous Coronary Intervention: The SMART-CHOICE Randomized Clinical Trial. JAMA - J. Am. Med. Assoc. 2019;321:2428-2437.

[33] Vranckx P, Valgimigli M, Jüni P, et al. Ticagrelor plus aspirin for 1 month, followed by ticagrelor monotherapy for 23 months vs aspirin plus clopidogrel or ticagrelor for 12 months, followed by aspirin monotherapy for 12 months after implantation of a drug-eluting stent: a multicentre, open-la. Lancet 2018;392:940-949.

[34] Franzone A, McFadden E, Leonardi S, et al. Ticagrelor Alone Versus Dual Antiplatelet Therapy From 1 Month After Drug-Eluting Coronary Stenting. J. Am. Coll. Cardiol. 2019;74:2223-2234.

[35] Watanabe H, Domei T, Morimoto T, et al. Effect of 1-Month Dual Antiplatelet Therapy Followed by Clopidogrel vs 12-Month Dual Antiplatelet Therapy on Cardiovascular and Bleeding Events in Patients Receiving PCI: The STOPDAPT-2 Randomized Clinical Trial. JAMA - J. Am. Med. Assoc. 2019;321:2414-2427.

[36] Yusuf S, Zhao F, Mehta SR, Chrolavicius S, Tognoni G, Fox KK. Effects of clopidogrel in addition to aspirin in patients with acute coronary syndromes without ST-segment elevation. N. Engl. J. Med. 2001;345:494-502.

[37] Mehta SR, Yusuf S, Peters RJG, et al. Effects of pretreatment with clopidogrel and aspirin followed by long-term therapy in patients undergoing percutaneous coronary intervention: The PCI-CURE study. Lancet 2001;358:527-533.

[38] Wiviott SD, Braunwald E, McCabe CH, et al. Prasugrel versus clopidogrel in patients with acute coronary syndromes. N. Engl. J. Med. 2007;357:2001-15. Available at: http://www.ncbi.nlm.nih.gov/pubmed/17982182.

[39] Wallentin L, Becker RC, Budaj A, et al. Ticagrelor versus clopidogrel in patients with acute coronary syndromes. N. Engl. J. Med. 2009;361:1045-1057. Available at: http://www.nejm.org/doi/abs/10.1056/NEJMoa0904327.

[40] Hahn JY, Song Y Bin, Oh JH, et al. 6-month versus 12-month or longer dual antiplatelet therapy after percutaneous coronary intervention in patients with acute coronary syndrome (SMART-DATE): a randomised, open-label, non-inferiority trial. Lancet 2018;391:1274-1284.

[41] Kim BK, Hong SJ, Cho YH, et al. Effect of Ticagrelor Monotherapy vs Ticagrelor with Aspirin on Major Bleeding and Cardiovascular Events in Patients with Acute Coronary Syndrome: The TICO Randomized Clinical Trial. JAMA - J. Am. Med. Assoc. 2020;323:2407-2416.

[42] Fiedler KA, Maeng M, Mehilli J, et al. Duration of Triple Therapy in Patients Requiring Oral Anticoagulation After Drug-Eluting Stent Implantation: The ISAR-TRIPLE Trial. J. Am. Coll. Cardiol. 2015;65:1619-1629. Available at: http://www.ncbi.nlm.nih.gov/pubmed/25908066.

[43] Dewilde WJM, Oirbans T, Verheugt FWA, et al. Use of clopidogrel with or without aspirin in patients taking oral anticoagulant therapy and undergoing percutaneous coronary intervention: An open-label, randomised, controlled trial. Lancet 2013;381:1107-1115.

[44] Cannon CP, Bhatt DL, Oldgren J, et al. Dual Antithrombotic Therapy with Dabigatran after PCI in Atrial Fibrillation. N. Engl. J. Med. 2017;377:1513-1524.

[45] Gibson CM, Mehran R, Bode C, et al. Prevention of Bleeding in Patients with Atrial Fibrillation Undergoing PCI. N. Engl. J. Med. 2016;375:2423-2434.

[46] Lopes RD, Heizer G, Aronson R, et al. Antithrombotic Therapy after Acute Coronary Syndrome or PCI in Atrial Fibrillation. N. Engl. J. Med. 2019;380:1509-1524.

[47] Vranckx P, Valgimigli M, Eckardt L, et al. Edoxaban-based versus vitamin K antagonist-based antithrombotic regimen after successful coronary stenting in patients with atrial fibrillation (ENTRUST-AF PCI): a randomised, open-label, phase 3b trial. Lancet 2019;394:1335-1343.

[48] Gargiulo G, Goette A, Tijssen J, et al. Safety and efficacy outcomes of double vs. triple antithrombotic therapy in patients with atrial fibrillation following percutaneous coronary intervention: A systematic review and meta-analysis of non-Vitamin K antagonist oral anticoagulant-based randomized clinical trials. Eur. Heart J. 2019;40:3757-3767.

[49] Borre ED, Goode A, Raitz G, et al. Predicting Thromboembolic and Bleeding Event Risk in Patients with Non-Valvular Atrial Fibrillation: A Systematic Review. Thromb. Haemost. 2018;118:2171-2187.

[50] Byrne RA. Randomized Trial of COBRA PzF Stenting to REDUCE Duration of Triple Therapy (COBRA-REDUCE). In: Presented at TCT 2020.

[51] Mehran R. The XIENCE Short DAPT Program: XIENCE 90/28 - Evaluating the Safety of 3-month and 1-month DAPT in HBR Patients. In: Presented at TCT 2020.

[52] Kirtane AJ. EVOLVE Short DAPT: A Single Arm Study of 3-Month DAPT in Patients at High Bleeding Risk Treated with a Bioabsorbable Polymer- Based Everolimus-Eluting Stent. In: Presented at TCT 2019.

[53] Windecker S, Latib A, Kedhi E, et al. Polymer-based or polymer-free stents in patients at high bleeding risk. N. Engl. J. Med. 2020;382:1208-1218.

[54] Varenne O, Cook S, Sideris G, et al. Drug-eluting stents in elderly patients with coronary artery disease (SENIOR): a randomised single-blind trial. Lancet 2018;391:41-50.

Chapter 2

Percutaneous Coronary Intervention in Diabetic Patients

Carolina Espejo Paeres, Breda Hennessey, Manel Sabaté and Pilar Jimenez-Quevedo

Abstract

Cardiovascular disease (CVD) is responsible for 30% of deaths worldwide and is the leading cause of premature mortality in patients with diabetes mellitus (DM). One of the main contributors to the increased atherothrombotic risk in DM patients relates to their pro- inflammatory and prothrombotic status that involves abnormalities in endothelial and vascular smooth muscle cells, in platelet function and the coagulation cascade. The characteristics of CAD in diabetic patients is distinctive and infers an increased risk. Likewise, CAD in diabetics is characterised by being diffuse, affecting the left main stem more frequently, involving multiple vessels, and also affecting the distal coronary tree. Percutaneous coronary intervention in diabetics has been shown to have less favourable long-term clinical outcomes, compared to non-diabetics. With the advent of improved stent designs and antiplatelet drugs; the percutaneous coronary intervention (PCI) results have improved in the diabetic population. However, one of the main determinants of poorer outcomes in DM is the progression of atherosclerosis, which is more pronounced in diabetics and remains the primary cause of cardiac events at one year follow up after percutaneous revascularisation. Whilst new generation of drug-eluting stents has narrowed the gap between surgery and PCI in diabetic patients, coronary artery bypass grafting (CABG) remains the gold standard in diabetics with diffuse multivessel coronary artery disease.

Keywords: diabetes mellitus, coronary artery bypass grafting, percutaneous coronary intervention, antiplatelet drugs, drug-eluting stents

1. Introduction

The prevalence of diabetes mellitus has increased exponentially, from 108 million in 1980 to 422 million worldwide in 2014 [1]. Cardiovascular diseases (CVDs) constitute the number one cause of mortality globally, representing 30% of all global deaths [2]. Cardiovascular disease is the leading cause of morbidity and premature mortality in patients with diabetes mellitus (DM) [3–6]. A meta-analysis of 102 prospective studies (The Emerging Risk Factor Collaboration) showed that DM in general, confers an increased risk for developing vascular disease compared to non-diabetic patients [7]. DM increases the risk of coronary heart disease, stroke, and peripheral arterial disease by between two and four-fold. The increased risk is independent of, and additional to other cardiovascular risk factors [7–10].

It has been reported that between 20 and 30% of patients with coronary artery disease have known DM, and up to 70% have newly detected DM or impaired glucose tolerance [11]. Importantly, the risk of myocardial infarction (MI) is three to five times higher in type 2 DM. A diabetic patient with no history of MI has the same long-term risk as a non-DM subject with a past history of MI [12]. For these reasons, DM is considered to be a "coronary heart disease equivalent" [13]. The anatomical pattern of coronary artery disease (CAD) in patients with DM influences the prognosis [11]. The extension of CAD in diabetic patients exhibits distinctive characteristics that infer an increased risk. Likewise, CAD in diabetics is characterised by being diffuse, affecting the left main stem more frequently, involving multiple vessels, and also affecting the distal coronary tree [14]. CAD typically progresses more rapidly in diabetic compared with non-diabetics [15]. Furthermore, patients with DM have more associated comorbidities, such as peripheral artery disease, cerebrovascular disease or chronic kidney disease, which influence outcomes after coronary revascularisation [11].

The indications for myocardial revascularisation, for both symptomatic and prognostic reasons, were the same in patients with or without DM [16]. The anatomical pattern in which diabetes affects patients, combined with an increased risk of stent failure (restenosis and stent thrombosis), in conjunction with the "Prothrombotic State" that characterised these patients, resulted in poorer outcomes following revascularisation in general. However, it is particularly evident following percutaneous revascularisation.

Three randomised clinical trials compared percutaneous coronary intervention (PCI) vs. coronary artery bypass graft surgery in patients with DM, using mainly first-generation drug-eluting stents (DES) [11]. With this in mind, safety concerns following PCI have surfaced, specifically with the use of first-generation DES, as diabetes has emerged as an independent predictor of stent thrombosis (ST) [17]. Recently, new generation DES platforms were designed and have demonstrated improved safety outcomes, compared to the first generation. Thus, coronary artery bypass grafting has been the revascularisation treatment recommended in diabetics with multivessel disease.

Although the advent of drug-eluting stents has narrowed the gap between surgery and the percutaneous treatment, the former remains the gold standard in diabetics with diffuse coronary artery disease.

One of the main determinants of poor outcomes in DM is the progression of atherosclerosis, which is more pronounced in diabetics and remains the main cause of cardiac events at one year follow up, after percutaneous revascularisation. This review focuses on all the aforementioned issues, which affect diabetic patients, as well as any updates to the current evidence regarding the different modalities of revascularisation in this special population.

2. Vascular abnormalities and atherothrombotic risk in diabetic patients

DM is linked to an increased atherothrombotic risk. In fact, diabetics with coronary artery disease suffer a higher rate of recurrence following their index MI [18]. Atherothrombotic disease is accelerated in subjects with both type 1 and type 2 diabetes, with diverse underlying mechanisms, despite the common characteristic of hyperglycaemia. The main feature of type 2 DM is insulin resistance, which precedes the development of hyperglycaemia [19]. Contrastingly, in type 1 diabetes, hyperglycaemia is the dominant feature with insulin resistance appearing at later stages, in patients who develop renal disease [20].

One of the main contributors to the increased atherothrombotic risk in DM patients relates to their pro- inflammatory and prothrombotic status that involves abnormalities in endothelial and vascular smooth muscle cells, in platelet function and the coagulation cascade. Endothelial dysfunction in diabetics is characterised by a decrease in nitric oxide (NO), and also by an increase in the synthesis of vasoconstrictor prostanoids and endothelin [21]. Hyperglycaemia decreases endothelium-derived NO via multiple mechanisms, including the intracellular production of advanced glycation end-products (AGEs) and free radical formation [22, 23]. Furthermore, hyperglycaemia also produces an increase in the concentration in plasma of vasoconstrictors, such as endothelin, which is related to both the incidence of inflammation and smooth-muscle contraction and growth. Other metabolic disorders known to occur in diabetes including an increase in the circulating levels of free fatty acid, an increase in the production of free radicals or an exacerbation of dyslipidaemia, may also impair the endothelial function [24–26]. On the other hand, hyperinsulinemia [27] also plays an important role in the pathophysiological mechanisms that may contribute towards vascular disease in diabetic patients. The concentration in plasma of vasoconstrictors, such as endothelin, increases after administration of insulin to healthy subjects and patients with type 2 diabetes [28–31]. This phenomenon may be related to both the incidence of inflammation and smooth-muscle contraction and growth. In addition, hyperinsulinemia is a potent mitogen for restenosis, as it stimulates the proliferation and migration of smooth cells [32]. Previous studies have demonstrated that hyperinsulinaemia enhances the secretion of insulin during the oral glucose tolerance test, and is a predictor of restenosis after balloon angioplasty and stent implantation [33–35].

Platelets are also affected in diabetic patients. Both insulin resistance and hyperglycaemia contribute to a prothrombotic state by exerting several salient effects on both coagulation and platelet function. The effects of insulin resistance on platelet function is related to intra-cytosolic calcium levels, a mediator of platelet activation. Whilst insulin decreases the intra-cellular concentration of calcium in platelets from insulin-sensitive subjects *in vivo* and *in vitro*, it appears to increase the intra-platelet calcium concentrations in the insulin-resistant state, promoting platelet aggregation and activation [36]. Platelets obtained from diabetic subjects showed both increased adhesiveness and an exaggerated aggregation following activation [24]. In addition, reduced responsiveness of diabetic patients to antiplatelet therapy has been documented [14]. The overall picture of platelet abnormalities in DM results in the hypersensitivity of diabetic platelets to agonists. In fact, platelets in diabetic subjects appear to be in an activated state even in the absence of vascular injury, and they respond more frequently even to sub threshold stimuli. It has been shown that there is greater expression of the fibrinogen-binding glycoprotein IIb/IIIa receptor, which constitutes the final common pathway of platelet activation and allows for cross-linking of individual platelets by fibrinogen molecules and formation of thrombus [15]. Finally, there is also impairment of the coagulation cascade. Insulin resistance gives rise to increased levels of the fibrinolytic inhibitor Plasminogen Activator Inhibitor-1 (PAI-1), and hyperglycaemia induces the enhancement of thromboxane A2 production and an increase in factor VII and anti-thrombin III production [24–26].

The alteration in platelet function is especially relevant in diabetics patients treated percutaneously, as it may affect the response to antiplatelet treatment. Although, clopidogrel response variability is a multifactorial process, the mechanisms above explain why dual antiplatelet regimen with ASA and clopidogrel presents important limitations in diabetic patients. The main mechanisms in this patient cohort that explain poor response to dual antiplatelet therapy in diabetes mellitus are antiplatelet resistance and clopidogrel response variability. Variability in antiplatelet effects following clopidogrel therapy is present in both the acute and the chronic phases of therapy [37]. Of note, diabetics requiring insulin are those who persist with the highest platelet reactivity, despite dual antiplatelet therapy [37]. This antiplatelet variability has clinical implications, such as increased rates of coronary stent thrombosis and recurrent ischaemic events after PCI in poor clopidogrel responders. Among the clinical factors involved in clopidogrel variability, diabetes mellitus has been associated with a greater prevalence of poor responsiveness [38]. Overall, the persistence of elevated platelet reactivity and reduced response to aspirin and clopidogrel therapy enhances the atherothrombotic risk of DM patients. Multiple causes have been implicated in these observations. Poor glycaemic control is an important cause of increased platelet reactivity. Hyperglycaemia leads to non-enzymatic glycation of platelet glycoproteins, causing changes in their structure and conformation, as well as alterations of membrane lipid dynamics. This may explain why platelet reactivity can be reduced with tight control of glucose levels [39].

The introduction of new regimens and antiplatelet agents may improve and overcome the variability in the response to clopidogrel. The P2Y12 inhibitors, with a more uniform and potent effect, have recently been evaluated. Prasugrel is a P2Y12 inhibitor of the third generation, with more potent and less variable antiplatelet effects compared to clopidogrel [40]. The TRITON-TIMI 38 (TRial to Assess Improvement in Therapeutic Outcomes by Optimising Platelet InhibitioN with Prasugrel-Thrombolysis in Myocardial Infarction) trial showed significantly reduced rates of ischaemic events, including stent thrombosis, in patients presenting with acute coronary syndromes undergoing PCI treated with prasugrel compared to clopidogrel [41]. In the subgroup analyses of diabetes population (n = 3146) the greatest risk reduction (rate of primary endpoint, defined as death from cardiovascular causes, non-fatal MI or non-fatal stroke) was observed in 12.2% of the diabetics treated with prasugrel vs. 17.0% in diabetic patients on clopidogrel with 30% relative risk reduction. Importantly, prasugrel was not associated with an increased risk of major bleedings compared to clopidogrel in these patients [42]. The functional impact of prasugrel versus clopidogrel, specifically in diabetic patients, was evaluated in the OPTIMUS-3 study. In this prospective, randomised, double-blind, crossover study, the standard-dose prasugrel was associated with greater platelet inhibition and better response profiles during both the loading and maintenance periods, when compared with double-dose clopidogrel [43].

On the other hand, ticagrelor, has a faster onset and offset of action and achieves higher inhibition of platelet aggregation compared to clopidogrel. In the RESPOND trial [44] Ticagrelor therapy overcomes nonresponsiveness to clopidogrel, and its antiplatelet effect is the same in responders and non-responders. The phase III Study of Platelet Inhibition and Patient Outcomes (PLATO) trial randomised acute coronary syndrome patients (n = 18,624) to receive either ticagrelor (180 mg loading dose followed by 90 mg twice daily) or clopidogrel (300–600 mg loading dose followed by 75 mg daily). In a predefined subgroup analysis of diabetic patients (n = 4662) there was a non-significant reduction of the primary endpoint [14.1% vs. 16.2%; HR 0.88 (0.76–1.03)], while no difference in major bleeding rates was found [14.1% vs. 14.8%; HR = 0.95 (0.81–1.12)] [45]. The recommendations from the recent ESC guidelines for the selection of antithrombotic therapy in diabetic patients with an acute coronary syndromes in patients presenting without persistent ST-segment elevation, state that the therapy should not differ from those without diabetes [46].

Phase III trial data on the use of factor-Xa inhibition direct oral anticoagulants for treatment of ACS has emerged. The APPRAISE-2 (Apixaban for Prevention of

Acute Ischemic Events) resulted in early termination of the study, due to an increase in Thrombolysis in Myocardial Infarction (TIMI) major bleeding in apixaban 5 mg bid (1.3%) compared with placebo (0.5%). There was no improvement in the composite of cardiovascular death, MI, or ischemic stroke with apixaban compared with placebo. Similarly, the ATLAS ACS 2-TIMI 51 (Anti Xa Therapy to Lower Cardiovascular Events in Addition to ASA with or without Thienopyridine Therapy in Subjects with Acute Coronary Syndrome—Thrombolysis in Myocardial Infarction) study had a significant increase in major bleeding with their respective Factor Xa inhibitors compared with dual antiplatelet therapy. It was noted however, in the primary analysis of the combined dosing arms, rivaroxaban (combined dose arms) reduced the composite of cardiovascular death, MI, or stroke compared with placebo (8.9% versus 10.7%, respectively). In a secondary analysis of the efficacy and safety of rivaroxaban (2.5 or 5 mg bid) compared with placebo in a pooled subset of ACS patients from the ATLAS ACS-TIMI 46 (phase II) and ATLAS ACS 2-TIMI 51 (phase III) trials [47] showed that the addition of rivaroxaban to aspirin reduced a composite of cardiovascular death, myocardial infarction, and stroke versus aspirin alone, primarily by a reduction in the risk of myocardial infarction. However, the combined rivaroxaban dose groups were associated with higher rates of non-CABG TIMI major bleeding. The use of these strategies specifically in diabetic patients remains under investigation. In the stable cardiovascular disease setting, the Cardiovascular OutcoMes for People using Anticoagulation StrategieS (COMPASS) trial [48] investigated very low-dose rivaroxaban (2.5 mg b.i.d.) in combination with aspirin vs. aspirin alone or rivaroxaban 5 mg b.i.d. alone. Those assigned to rivaroxaban (2.5 mg twice daily) plus aspirin had better cardiovascular outcomes and more major bleeding events than those assigned to aspirin alone. Greater absolute risk reductions were seen in high-risk patients, including those with diabetes.

3. Percutaneous revascularisation in diabetic patients

Since its inception, the use of percutaneous transluminal balloon angioplasty (BA) to treat coronary stenosis, diabetics have shown less favourable long-term clinical outcomes, compared to non-diabetics. Diabetes mellitus has been identified as an independent predictor of restenosis. In fact, the restenosis rate following BA in diabetics ranges between 35% and 71%, which is much higher than seen in the general population (30–35%) [49]. In addition, the pattern of restenosis is more severe, as these patients typically show more proliferative and occlusive types of restenosis. The main contributor to the restenosis process following plain BA is negative remodelling (i.e., vessel shrinkage) [50] that accounts for 73% of lumen reduction after balloon angioplasty, while plaque burden contributes 27% [51].

Coronary stenting was able to reduce the occurrence of restenosis, not only in general population but also in diabetic patients [52]. Two pivotal randomised controlled trials demonstrated the beneficial effects of stenting as compared to BA, the STRESS and the BENESTENT trials [53, 54]. The analysis of diabetic patients in these two trials revealed a significant reduction in restenosis rate (STRESS: stent 32%, balloon 42%; p = 0.046; BENESTENT: stent 22%, balloon 42%; p = 0.02) and clinical outcomes improvement at 6 months and at 4 years follow-up (including cardiac death, non-fatal MI and the need for repeat revascularization) [55]. Despite these results, restenosis rate remained higher in diabetics compared to non-diabetics. In a meta-analysis [56] of 16 studies, after stent implantation angiographic restenosis (defined as ≥50% diameter stenosis at follow-up) occurred in 550 of 2672 (20.6%) of non-diabetics as compared to 130 of 418 (31.1%) of diabetic patients

($p < 0.001$). The authors identified, among other factors, insulin treatment in type 2 diabetes, a marker of disease duration and severity, as an independent predictor of restenosis. The prevailing mechanism of restenosis after stenting is accelerated intimal hyperplasia which is especially exaggerated in diabetic patients [57]. Thus, the development of drug-eluting stent (DES) to tackle this mechanism of restenosis directly was a revolutionary development in this field. In this regard, the subgroup analysis of the two pivotal randomised trial, which evaluated the efficacy of first generation DES (Cypher® stent; Cordis, Johnson & Johnson, Warren, NJ, USA and Taxus® stent; Boston Scientific, Natick, MA, USA) showed positive results in terms of restenosis rates and in MACE [58, 59].

In the SIRIUS trial (Sirolimus-coated Bx Velocity balloon-expandable stent in the treatment of patients with de novo coronary artery lesions) [60] a total of 1058 patients were randomised to either SES or BMS for the treatment of de novo coronary stenosis. The primary endpoint was target vessel failure (cardiac death, myocardial infarction and target vessel revascularisation [TVR]) at 9-month follow-up. The diabetes subgroup analysis of the SIRIUS trial included 279 patients, 131 receiving SES and 148 receiving BMS [61]. In this subgroup of patients, SES implantation demonstrated favourable results with significant reductions in restenosis rates (in-lesion 50% for BMS vs. 17% for SES), and in MACE (25% for BMS vs. 9.2% for SES). The TAXUS IV trial [62] enrolled 1326 patients that were randomised to PES or BMS for the treatment of de novo coronary stenosis. The primary endpoint was ischaemia driven TVR and the incidence of cardiac death, and MI at one year. Overall, the PES group showed a significant reduction in the occurrence of the primary endpoint (TVR 7.4% vs. 20.9%, $p = 0.0008$). The study included 155 diabetic patients (32% of the total population) and 33% of the diabetics were insulin-dependent DM. In this subgroup, the use of PES significantly reduced the risk of binary restenosis (70% reduction of in-segment restenosis). This reduction was also observed in insulin-dependent DM subjects (42.9% for BMS vs. 7.7% for PES, $p = 0.007$).

The DIABETES (Diabetes and Sirolimus-Eluting Stent) trial [63] was the first randomised multicentre controlled trial specifically designed to assess the efficacy of SES vs. BMS in diabetics. This study included 160 diabetic patients, 80 of whom received BMS, while 80 were treated with SES. Late lumen loss assessed by QCA at 9-month follow-up was the primary endpoint. The SES treated group showed a significant reduction of late lumen loss (relative reduction 87%). The study considered a sub-randomisation, according to the type of anti-diabetic treatment and the SES benefit was independent from diabetic status. This benefit was maintained up to 5-year follow-up [64]. Subsequently, 3 other randomised trials also designed for diabetic patients (SCORPIUS [65, 66], DESSERT [67] and DECODE [68]) have corroborated the same positive results of SES in reducing neointimal proliferation to mid and long-term. A meta-analysis of all available data in diabetics treated with PCI [69] demonstrated the benefit of DES in terms of restenosis and target lesion revascularisation.

Finally, other studies compared both DES in terms of efficacy (**Table 1**). The SIRTAX (SIRolimus versus pacliTAXel-eluting stents) trial [70] and the ISAR (In-Stent Angiographic Restenosis)-DIABETES trial [71] showed that SES in diabetics had lower MACE and lower late lumen loss compared with PES. The efficacy of new generation DES has also been evaluated. The everolimus-eluting stent (EES) has been tested against PES in the SPIRIT IV and V trial. In the subgroup analyses of the SPIRIT IV [72] EES compared with PES showed no difference in target lesion failure (6.4% vs. 6.9%, respectively, $p = 0.80$) or any of its components was present among diabetic patients, regardless of insulin use. In contrast, in the SPIRIT V

Trial	Type of study	Type of stent	N	Primary endpoint	Primary outcomes
SIRTAX [90]	Single-centre, controlled, single-blind trial	SES vs. PES#	250	MACE (cardiac death, myocardial infarction and ischemia-driven target lesion revascularisation)	The primary endpoint was significantly lower in the SES group. The difference between SES and PES stents was more pronounced in the DM patients.
ISAR-DIABETES [91]	P, NI trial	SES vs. PES in diabetics	250	In-segment late lumen loss (non-inferiority margin 0.16mm)	In-segment late luminal loss was greater in the paclitaxel-stent group than in the sirolimus-stent group (P=0.002)
SPIRIT V DIABETIC [92]	P, single-blind, R.	EES vs. PES in diabetics	324	In-stent late lumen loss at 8 months	EES was superior to PES for in-stent late loss at 9 months however, clinical endpoints were similar between the two groups.
ESSENCE DIABETESbis [92]	P, M, R	EES vs. SES in diabetics	300	In-segment late lumen loss at 8 months	Everolimus-eluting stents were noninferior to sirolimus-eluting stents in reducing Late lumen loss:.
ENDEAVOR IV [93]	P, R (1:1), single-blind, controlled trial	ZES vs. PES #	477	Target vessel failure at 9 months	A trend towards higher in-stent late loss with ZES as compared to PES, but with comparable clinical outcomes at 1-year follow-up.
RESOLUTE [94]	M, NI trial	ZES vs. EES #	538	Target vessel failure at 12 months	ZES was demonstrated to be non-inferior to EES
LEADERS [95]	M, assessor-blind, NI	BES vs. SES#	414	Composite endpoint*	The primary endpoint was comparable in diabetic patients

SES: sirolimus-eluting stent; BMS: bare metal stent; PES: paclitaxel-eluting stent; DM: diabetes mellitus; EES: everolimus-eluting stent; ZES: zotarolimus-eluting stent; BES: biolimus-eluting stent; MACE: major adverse cardiac events; TVF: target vessel failure; TVR: target vessel revascularisation; P: prospective; NI: non-inferiority trial, R: randomised; M: multicenter.
Composite endpoint of cardiac death, myocardial infarction and clinically-driven target vessel revascularisation at 9 months.
#*Diabetic subgroup.*

Table 1.
Randomised controlled trials comparing drug-eluting stent vs. drug-eluting stents in diabetic patients.

Diabetic Study Everolimus-eluting stent was superior to PES for in-stent late loss at 9 months, however, clinical endpoints were similar between the two groups [73]. Interestingly no stent thromboses (Academic Research Consortium definite and probable) were seen at 1 year with EES, compared with 2 of 104 (2%) with PES (P = 0.11). The efficacy of the zotarolimus-eluting stent (ZES) has been assessed in the Endeavour IV trial against PES [74] and the Resolute™ [75] stent a new generation ZES against EES. In these studies, ZES was comparable with PES and non-inferior to EES. Finally, the biolimus-eluting stent (BES) has been compared to SES in the LEADERS all-comer trial. BES appeared to be non-inferior to SES with regard to the primary endpoint in the subgroup of diabetics [76].

The effectiveness of different DES platforms has been addressed in the Swedish Angiography and Angioplasty Registry (SCAAR) [77]. Data on restenosis from 2004 and 2008 was collected. Four DES types qualified for inclusion. In total, 35,478 DES were implanted at 22,962 procedures in 19,004 patients and 1807 restenosis events were reported over a mean 29-month follow-up. In the entire study population, the restenosis rate per stent was 3.5% after 1 year and 4.9% after 2 years. The adjusted risk of restenosis was higher in patients with DM, compared to patients without DM (relative risk [RR]: 1.23, 95% confidence interval [CI]: 1.10 to 1.37). In patients with DM, restenosis was twice as frequent with the ZES stent compared with that in SES and PES types.

Another important aspect in the use of DES is the safety, especially in diabetic patients. Safety of DES mainly refers to the incidence of ST, MI or death during follow-up. Diabetes has been identified as an independent predictor of ST in many registries with the use of first-generation DES (SES and PES) [17, 78]. In a large multicentric registry 66 of more than 15,000 patients treated with SES, the overall incidence of stent thrombosis at 1 year was 0.87% and the most potent independent predictor of thrombosis was the insulin-dependent DM [78]. Diabetic patients, as mentioned previously, exhibit specific pathophysiological factors as well as unfavourable angiographic parameters, which confers an especially high risk of thrombosis.

A Swedish Registry (SCAAR) compared diabetic patients treated with DES to those treated with BMS. The median follow-up was 2.5 years. This study included 4754 patients who received at least one DES and 4956 patients that received only bare metal stents (BMS) at the index procedure. The study showed that restenosis was halved by DES in diabetic patients with stable or unstable coronary disease, compared with BMS [RR, 0.50 (95% CI, 0.35–0.70)] and was associated with a higher adjusted RR of MI, [RR 5.03 (95% CI, 4.25–5.97)] [79]. Similar results were observed in a meta-analysis of individual patient data from four randomised trials reporting on the use of SES in diabetics [80]. This meta-analysis included 583 patients (SES vs. BMS; median follow-up of 4.2 years). There was a significant reduction in the overall hazard of MACE (hazard ratio, [HR] 0.48, 95% confidence interval [CI] 0.36–0.63, P < 0.001) with SES. The overall hazard of death (HR 0.91, 95% CI 0.59–1.41, P = 0.68), as well as death or MI (HR 0.77, 95% CI 0.54–1.09, P = 0.14), was not significantly different between the groups. No significant differences were observed regarding ST (HR 0.50, 95% CI 0.15–1.69, P = 0.26) [80]. Reassuring data also comes from the Massachusetts Data Analysis Registry that included 6008 diabetics treated between April 2003 and September 2004. After propensity score-matched risk analysis, the use of DES was associated with a significantly lower rate of death, MI and TVR [52].

New generation EES stent showed a safety benefit as compared to PES in the Spirit V- diabetic randomised trial at 1 year; the composite of death and MI was reduced by EES (9.6% vs. 3.7%; p = 0.04) as well as the thrombosis rate (1.9% vs. 0%; p = ns) [73].

Data concerning safety of BES in diabetics comes from a sub-study from the LEADERS trial. Among insulin-dependent diabetics, the rate of all-cause death and cardiac death was 0% after BES implantation, compared to 9.1% and 6.5% respectively, after SES implantation at 12 months follow-up ($p < 0.01$) [76].

Finally, the Resolute™ stent showed a higher incidence of definite ST at 1-year follow-up, compared to EES (1.2% vs. 0.3%; <0.01) in the all-comer RESOLUTE trial [81].

4. Multivessel disease in diabetics

Based on the current evidence, coronary artery bypass graft (CABG) is the treatment of choice for diabetic patients with multivessel disease [82]. However, since the inception of percutaneous coronary intervention, numerous trials have been designed to evaluate the efficacy of PCI versus CABG in patients with multivessel disease. In the following section, we will discuss the various trials that have compared surgical revascularisation to percutaneous intervention, beginning with balloon angioplasty and continuing to the modern DES era.

4.1 Trials comparing CABG and BA

Four trials designed to compare the efficacy of CABG versus BA have reported data on the subgroup of patients with diabetes mellitus: the EAST study, the BARI study, the CABRI trial and the RITA trial (**Table 2**) [83–86]. The only study that showed a significant benefit in survival of diabetic patients treated with CABG compared with BA, was the BARI trial. On the basis of these results, a clinical alert to US physicians from the National Heart, Lung, and Blood Institute, was published in Circulation 1995 and concluded that CABG should be the preferred treatment for patients with diabetes on drug or insulin therapy, who have multivessel coronary artery disease and require a first coronary revascularisation procedure.

Trial	Inclusion/exclusion criteria	Primary endpoint	Number diabetics included	F-U	Primary endpoint in DM
BARI [80]	Angina or severe ischemia, CAD amenable for BA or CABG	10-year survival	CABG DM: 180 BA DM: 173	7.8	PTCA 45.5% vs. CABG 57.8%, p = 0.025).
EAST [79]	MV CAD, no previous Rev; no LMS stenosis, no CTO, no LVEF ≤25%	3-year death, MI	CABG: 41 BA: 49	8-10.5	CABG: 75.5% BA: 60.1% *p*= 0.23
CABRI [82]	Age ≤76, MV CAD + clinical evident ischemia; no previous Rev, LMS stenosis, LVEF ≤25%, stroke, HF	Mortality	CABG: 60 BA: 64	4	CABG: 12.5% BA: 22.6% *p*= 0.01
RITA [81]	>50-70% coronary stenosis SA or UA, *de novo* single or MV CAD suitable for BA or CABG	5-year death, non fatal MI	CABG: 33 BA: 29	6.5	CABG: 16% BA: 17% *p*= 0.64

Table 2.
Randomised Controlled Trials comparing Balloon angioplasty versus CABG in patients with multivessel disease.

4.2 Trials comparing CABG versus PCI with bare metal stents

There are four randomised trial that compared the outcomes from bypass surgery versus coronary stenting in patients with multivessel disease: the ARTS, the AWESOME trial, the SOS and the ERACI II trial. Only the first two trials analysed the diabetic subgroup separately, and neither showed any survival benefit. The ARTS (Arterial Revascularisation Therapy Study) trial reported a reduced event-free survival at 1 year in diabetics treated with stenting, as compared with those treated with CABG (63.4% vs. 84.4%, $p = 0.001$) [87]. This difference was largely due to a significant increase in repeat revascularisation in the stent group. Of note, the rate of complete revascularisation in patients who underwent PCI was only (70.5%) compared with those who had CABG (84.1%). Conversely, the rate of death and MI in diabetic were similar between groups (6.7% vs. 3.1%, $p = 0.29$ and 6.3% vs. 3.1%, $p = 0.29$, respectively). In addition, a trend towards an increase in the rate of cerebrovascular events was observed in the CABG group (1.8% vs. 6.3%, $p = 0.009$). At five years, there was no significant difference in mortality between the two groups. However, it was noted, that the rate of myocardial infarction was highest in the BMS arm, compared with CABG arm (11.0% vs. 5.2%). The AWESOME trial (Angina With Extremely Serious Operative Mortality Evaluation Trial) randomised 454 patients with multivessel disease to either CABG or stenting. Among diabetics, the respective CABG and PCI 36-month survival rates were comparable (72% for CABG vs. 81% for PCI) [88]. A collaborative analysis of data from ten randomised trials to compare the effectiveness of CABG with PCI (six trials used balloon angioplasty and four trials used with bare-metal stents), in patients with multivessel disease, showed that patients with diabetes (CABG, $n = 615$; PCI, $n = 618$), mortality was substantially lower in the CABG group than in the PCI group (HR 0.70, 0.56–0.87) [89].

In summary, despite these trials demonstrating a reduced need for subsequent revascularization following PCI with stents as compared to BA, the need for repeat revascularization remained significantly higher when compared to CABG in the diabetic population with multivessel disease. Moreover, the rate of myocardial infarction in diabetics was higher at long-term follow-up with the use of stents as compared to CABG. Thus, in the BMS era, revascularisation of diabetic patients with multivessel disease, CABG remained the first option of revascularization in patients suitable for surgery.

4.3 Trials comparing CABG and DES

The data available in the current era of DES comes from a combination of registry data, subgroup analysis from two randomised trials (the SYNTAX trial and the EXCEL trial) and two randomised trial performed specifically in diabetics patients. Beginning with the registry data, there are two multicentre registries that report data for diabetic patients treated with DES: the ERACI-3 and the ARTS 2 registries. Both registries compared a current cohort of patients with multivessel disease treated with drug-eluting stents with the historical cohort of patients from ERACI 2 and ARTS 1 trial respectively; treated with either CABG or conventional BM stenting. The ARTS 2 registry was a single arm trial that included 607 patients with multivessel disease treated with SES. The ARTS I and II studies included 367 diabetic patients (SES: 159, CABG: 96, and BMS: 112); at the 5-year follow up, the rate of major adverse cardiovascular and cerebrovascular events were significantly higher in patients treated with BMS (BMS 53.6% vs. CABG 23.4% vs. SES 40.5%; $p < 0.01$ for SES vs. BMS and SES vs. CABG). There was no significant difference in mortality among all 3 groups. There was an advantage of CABG over SES in reducing repeat revascularisation procedures; interestingly revascularisation rate of patients treated with SES at 5 years approached that of patients treated with BMS although remained significantly lower. This "catch-up" phenomenon was not apparent in the non-diabetic population [90].

In the diabetic subgroup of ERACI-3 registry [91], MACCE rates at 3 years were 36.2% in the DES arm, 43.6% in the BMS arm, and 30.8% in the CABG group ($p = 0.49$). Of the components of MACCE, TVR was the only one that differed significantly across the three groups: drug-eluting stent (21.3%), bare metal stent (38.5%), and CABG (15.4%); $p = 0.048$. There was a non-significant trend towards more death and non-fatal MI among diabetics treated with DES (19.1%), than in the bare metal stent (12.8%) or CABG (15.4%) cohort of ERACI-2. Sub-acute late-stent thrombosis occurred more frequently in DES-treated patients, compared with BMS patients ($P = 0.008$).

Another registry [92] compared DES implantation with off-pump CABG. This study addresses the effect of DES versus off-pump CABG, on 1-year outcome of diabetic patients with multivessel disease and critical stenosis, involving the proximal left anterior descending coronary artery, who underwent elective myocardial revascularisation. Following propensity score analysis, adjusting for baseline differences between the 2 cohorts, DES increased the risk of 12-month MACCE (HR 1.88, 95% CI, $p = 0.020$). This was due to the higher rate for repeat revascularisation in the DES group (19% vs. 5%, HR 2.05, 95% CI, $p = 0.001$). In contrast, there was no difference in the rate of the composite endpoints of death, MI, and stroke (DES group 13%, CABG group 12%; adjusted analysis, HR 0.80, 95% CI, $p = 0.40$). On the other hand, the New York registry [93] showed a trend towards improved outcomes in diabetic patients treated with CABG ($n = 3256$), compared with DES ($n = 2844$) (or for death or MI at 18 months 0.84, 95% CI 0.69–1.01; $p = 0.07$).

The SYNTAX (Synergy between percutaneous coronary intervention with TAXUS and cardiac surgery) trial randomly allocated 1800 patients with left main and/or 3-vessel coronary artery disease to PES implantation or CABG. In the subgroup of patients with DM ($n = 452$), MACCE rate was significantly higher at 1 year with PES than with CABG (26.0% vs. 14.2%; RR 1.83 [1.22–2.73]; $p = 0.003$), at the expense of higher repeat revascularisation with PES (6.4% vs. 20.3%; RR 3.18 [1.77–5.71]; $p < 0.001$). Safety endpoint (death, stroke or MI), as well as symptomatic graft occlusion or stent thrombosis rates were comparable between treatment arms. Of note, in patients with SYNTAX score > 33, death rate was significantly higher with PES (13.5% vs. 4.1%; $p = 0.04$) [94].

There are two randomised trials comparing DES and CABG in patients with diabetes. The CARDIA trial (Coronary Artery Revascularisation in Diabetes) [95] is a non-inferiority trial, comparing optimal PCI with modern CABG, as a revascularisation strategy for patients with diabetes who have multivessel or complex single-vessel coronary disease. The 1-year results of the CARDIA trial did not demonstrate the noninferiority of PCI versus CABG for revascularisation of diabetic patients. At 1 year, the primary endpoint (composite of death, non-fatal MI and non-fatal stroke) was comparable between arms (10.5% in CABG vs. 13.0% in PCI arm; $p = 0.39$), only further revascularisation was significantly higher in the PCI arm (2% vs. 11.8%; $p < 0.001$). Although this study was the first randomised trial that compared the two revascularisation strategies in diabetic patients, it was underpowered for the primary composite outcome. Therefore, further information on optimal strategies for coronary revascularisation in diabetic patients is needed.

The FREEDOM trial (Future Revascularisation Evaluation in Patients with Diabetes Mellitus: Optimal Management of Multivessel Disease) is a randomised trial, in which patients with diabetes and multivessel disease were randomly assigned to undergo multivessel PCI using DES versus bypass surgery and followed for up to 5 years. At 5 years follow-up, the primary outcome: a composite of death from any cause, nonfatal myocardial infarction, and nonfatal stroke occurred more frequently in the PCI group, compared with the CABG group (26.6% vs. 18.7%; $p = 0.005$). The benefit of CABG was driven by differences in rates of both myocardial infarction ($P < 0.001$) and death from any cause ($P = 0.049$). Cardiac death was not significant ($p = 0.12$). Stroke was more frequent in the CABG group than in the PCI group (2.4% vs. 5.2%; $p = 0.03$) [96].

The BARI 2 Diabetes (BARI 2D) [97] is a randomised, open, controlled, multicentre trial that compared optimal medical management with prompt revascularisation (PCI or CABG) in patients with type 2 DM and stable coronary disease. The primary endpoint was death from any cause. At 5-year follow-up, survival rate was comparable between groups (88%) with no difference in MACE or death. Patients treated with CABG showed much greater atherosclerotic burden and more lesions than the PCI stratum. Prompt revascularisation significantly reduced the MACE rate in those patients treated with CABG, largely because of a reduction in MI events, but not among those selected to undergo PCI as compared to optimal medical treatment. However, up to 42% of the patients allocated to optimal medical therapy required coronary revascularisation with PCI during the 5 years of follow-up [97].

A recent meta-analysis of 11 RCTs [98], involved 11,518 patients allocated to PCI or CABG. The 5-year all-cause mortality was 11.2% after PCI and 9.2% after CABG (HR 1.20, 95% CI 1.061.37; $P = 0.0038$). Among patients with DM, mortality rates were 15.7% in PCI and 10.1% in CABG (HR 1.44, 95% CI 1.201.74; $P = 0.0001$). Conversely, this difference was not found among non-diabetic patients.

There have been a number of studies comparing outcomes of CABG and PCI that involved the use of newer-generation DES. A large meta-analysis including 8095 patients with DM showed a significant reduction in MI, stent thrombosis, and MACE, with newer-generation everolimus-eluting stents, compared to first generation DES [99]. Data from the Randomised Comparison of Coronary Artery Bypass Surgery and Everolimus-Eluting Stent Implantation in the Treatment of Patients with Multivessel Coronary Artery Disease (BEST) study [100], showed that the outcomes were poorer in the PCI group, with the rate of the primary outcome of death, MI, or TVR at two years significantly higher (19.2 vs. 9.1%; $P = 0.007$). In a subgroup analysis of 505 patients with DM, in the Evaluation of XIENCE versus Coronary Artery Bypass Surgery for Effectiveness of Left Main Revascularisation (EXCEL) trial [101], the investigators reported the rate of the primary outcome of death, MI or stroke at three years occurred in 21.2% of patients in the PCI arm and 19.4% in the CABG arm (HR 1.04, 95% CI 0.70–1.55). In conclusion, is clear that we are yet to determine whether the newer generation DES will begin to narrow the divide favouring CABG for patients with DM and multivessel disease, and additionally, that further dedicated randomised control trials are needed.

5. The importance of atherosclerosis progression in the long-term outcome after myocardial revascularisation

Atherosclerotic coronary artery disease is a chronic condition that is not limited by revascularisation. The short and long-term outcomes in patients undergoing both percutaneous and surgical revascularisation, are not only determined by stent or graft failure, but also by atherosclerotic disease progression in other territories. A paucity of data exists regarding the impact of atherosclerosis progression on the outcome of patients after revascularisation, and this is particularly evident in patients with diabetes. The current data regarding atherosclerosis progression after percutaneous revascularisation is limited. One of the studies that address this issue was the study conducted by Cutlip et al. [102] This study included 1228 patients treated with BMS. The cumulative incidence of restenosis events, non-restenosis events, and the overall composite end point up to 5 years was evaluated. In this study, it was demonstrated that the events relating to restenosis increased during the first year, however there was a virtual absence of restenosis thereafter. On the other hand, the rate of non-restenosis events increased during the first year, in parallel to the restenosis events but continued to increase out to 5 years. The two factors that were independently associated with an increased risk of restenosis and non-restenosis events were diabetes and multivessel disease.

Zellweger et al. [103] studied the importance of 5-year coronary disease progression after successful DES stenting. This is a sub-study of the Basket trial and involved 428 consecutive patients randomised to drug-eluting versus bare-metal stents, with successful stenting documented by freedom from symptoms/events and non-ischaemic perfusion defects (PDs) after 6 months. Rest and stress scintigraphy scans were repeated after 60 months. Late events and new perfusion defects in areas remote from stented vessels were recorded. At 5 years follow-up, 37.1% of all events were due to remote MI, or remote repeat revascularisation. In addition, asymptomatic remote perfusion defect accounted for 37.5%. There is also information about the impact of atherosclerosis progression derived from large randomised trials comparing DES vs. BMS. In the 5-years of the SIRIUS (Sirolimus-Eluting Stent in De-Novo Native Coronary Lesions) trial, 28% of MI were located in non-target vessels. In addition, 64% in the SES group and the 42.% in the BMS group of all target vessel revascularisation were non performed in the target lesion [104]. In the 5-year TAXUS IV Treatment of De Novo Coronary Disease Using a Single Paclitaxel-Eluting Stent trial: 45% of all revascularisation in the PES group were due to non-target lesion TVR [105].

The progression of atherosclerosis in diabetics has been specifically assessed by Rozeman et al. [106]. This study included 248 patients (55 diabetics/193 non diabetics) and evaluated the percentage of arteries with new narrowing's at follow-up angiography following angioplasty. The authors observed that the percentage of new narrowing was more often in diabetic patients compared to non-diabetics (14.8 vs. 9.4%; $p = 0.03$) and particularly in the arteries previously treated with angioplasty (13.6 vs. 8.5; $p = 0.01$). The 5 year follow-up of the DIABETES (DIABETes and sirolimus-Eluting Stent) trial, showed that the need for new revascularisation in the SES group was due equally to restenosis and progression of atherosclerosis in other territories [64]. On the other hand, surgical revascularisation also have disease progression [107]. It has been described that the progression is primarily in the proximal segment before the anastomosis (74%) and the majority was proximal coronary occlusion (78%). This pattern of atherosclerosis progression may be mostly asymptomatic in patients with a patent graft and prevents future events due to plaque rupture in the proximal segment of the artery.

This data suggested that the clinical implication of atherosclerosis progression is different in the two-revascularisation strategies and negatively affects patients treated percutaneously, particularly after the first year of clinical follow-up. This has to be taken into account, when comparing long term results of stent implantation versus CABG in patients with multivessel disease. Improvements in both the stent platforms and the adoption of new drug coatings have improved the outcome of patients treated with PCI. However, it is critical, particularly in the diabetic population to improve the secondary prevention strategies to decrease the occurrence of events due to atherosclerosis progression.

6. Current recommendations for revascularisation in diabetics

Contemporary guidelines place emphasis on the long-term survival benefit conferred by CABG, for treatment of diabetics with multivessel disease. A clinician's judgement on the revascularisation strategy remains an important factor. Although PCI with DES has narrowed the gap with surgery, following the results of the FREEDOM trial in CABG-eligible diabetic patients multivessel disease, CABG remains the gold standard treatment [16, 96] (**Tables 3** and **4**).

Recommendations according to the extent of CAD	CABG		PCI	
	CLASS	LEVEL	CLASS	LEVEL
One vessel CAD				
Without proximal LAD stenosis	IIb	C	I	C
With proximal LAD stenosis	I	A	I	A
Two vessel CAD				
Without proximal LAD stenosis	IIb	C	I	C
With proximal LAD stenosis	I	B	I	C
Three vessel CAD				
With low disease complexity (SYNTAX score 0-22)	I	A	IIb	A
With intermediate or high disease complexity (SYNTAX score >22)	I	A	III	A
Left main CAD				
With low disease complexity (SYNTAX score 0-22)	I	A	I	A
With intermediate disease complexity (SYNTAX score 23-32)	I	A	IIa	A
With high disease complexity (SYNTAX score ≥ 33)	I	A	III	B

CABG = coronary artery bypass graft; CAD = coronary artery disease; DM = diabetes mellitus; LAD = left anterior descending coronary artery; PCI = percutaneous coronary intervention; SYNTAX = Synergy between Percutaneous Coronary Intervention with TAXUS and Cardiac Surgery.

Table 3.
Recommendations for the type of revascularization in patients with diabetes with stable coronary artery disease, suitable coronary anatomy for both procedures, and low predicted surgical mortality. Adapted from 2018 ESC/EACTS Guidelines on myocardial revascularization.

Recommendations	Class	Level
It is recommended that the same revascularisation techniques are implemented (e.g. the use of DES and the radial approach for PCI, and the use of the left internal mammary artery as the graft for CABG) in patients with and without DM.	I	A
It is recommended that renal function should be checked if patients are taking metformin immediately before angiography and that metformin should be withheld if renal function deteriorates.	I	C
Optimal medical therapy should be considered to be the preferred treatment in patients with CCS and DM unless there are uncontrolled ischaemic symptoms, large areas of ischaemia or significant left main or proximal LAD lesions.	IIa	B

CABG = coronary artery bypass graft; CCS = chronic coronary syndromes; DES = drug-eluting stent; DM = diabetes mellitus; EACTS = European Association for Cardio-Thoracic Surgery; ESC = European Society of Cardiology; LAD = left anterior descending coronary artery; PCI = percutaneous coronary intervention.

Table 4.
Recommendations for coronary revascularisation in patients with diabetes. Adapted from 2018 ESC/EACTS Guidelines on myocardial revascularization.

7. Conclusions

Diabetic patients are a very high-risk population. The unfavourable anatomy and the prothrombotic state contribute to the poor acute and midterm outcome following percutaneous revascularisations. With the advent of DES, improved stent designs and antiplatelet drugs; the rate of TLR and MACE has also improved in diabetic patients; however, it remains higher in comparison to non-diabetic patients. We have underestimated the impact of atherosclerosis progression in the appearance of late events after PCI, particularly in patients with diabetes. Whilst it is clearly evident that both aggressive secondary prevention and lifestyle modification are mandatory to alter the natural history of CAD in this group, the gold standard for diabetic patient with complex multivessel disease is surgical revascularisation.

Author details

Carolina Espejo Paeres[1], Breda Hennessey[1], Manel Sabaté[2] and Pilar Jimenez-Quevedo[1]*

1 Clinico San Carlos University Hospital, IdISSC, Madrid, Spain

2 University Hospital Clínic, Institut d'Investigacions Biomèdiques August Pi i Sunyer (IDIBAPS), Barcelona, Spain

*Address all correspondence to: patropjq@gmail.com

References

[1] Roglic G, World Health Organization, editors. Global report on diabetes. Geneva, Switzerland: World Health Organization; 2016. 86 p.

[2] Cardiovascular diseases [Internet]. [cited 2020 Sep 17]. Available from: https://www.who.int/westernpacific/health-topics/cardiovascular-diseases

[3] Nathan DM. Long-term complications of diabetes mellitus. N Engl J Med. 1993;328:1676-85.

[4] Read SH, McAllister DA, Colhoun HM, Farran B, Fischbacher C, Kerssens JJ, et al. Incident ischaemic stroke and Type 2 diabetes: trends in incidence and case fatality in Scotland 2004-2013. Diabet Med. 2018;35:99-106.

[5] Burrows NR, Li Y, Gregg EW, Geiss LS. Declining Rates of Hospitalization for Selected Cardiovascular Disease Conditions Among Adults Aged ≥35 Years With Diagnosed Diabetes, U.S., 1998-2014. Diabetes Care. 2018;41:293-302.

[6] Rawshani A, Rawshani A, Franzén S, Eliasson B, Svensson A-M, Miftaraj M, et al. Mortality and Cardiovascular Disease in Type 1 and Type 2 Diabetes. N Engl J Med. 2017;376:1407-18.

[7] Emerging Risk Factors Collaboration, Sarwar N, Gao P, Seshasai SRK, Gobin R, Kaptoge S, et al. Diabetes mellitus, fasting blood glucose concentration, and risk of vascular disease: a collaborative meta-analysis of 102 prospective studies. Lancet. 2010;375:2215-22.

[8] Brand FN, Abbott RD, Kannel WB. Diabetes, intermittent claudication, and risk of cardiovascular events. The Framingham Study. Diabetes. 1989;38:504-9.

[9] Stamler J, Vaccaro O, Neaton JD, Wentworth D. Diabetes, other risk factors, and 12-yr cardiovascular mortality for men screened in the Multiple Risk Factor Intervention Trial. Diabetes Care. 1993;16:434-44.

[10] Pahor M, Psaty BM, Furberg CD. New evidence on the prevention of cardiovascular events in hypertensive patients with type 2 diabetes. J Cardiovasc Pharmacol. 1998;32 Suppl 2:S18-23.

[11] Cosentino F, Grant PJ, Aboyans V, Bailey CJ, Ceriello A, Delgado V, et al. 2019 ESC Guidelines on diabetes, pre-diabetes, and cardiovascular diseases developed in collaboration with the EASDThe Task Force for diabetes, pre-diabetes, and cardiovascular diseases of the European Society of Cardiology (ESC) and the European Association for the Study of Diabetes (EASD). Eur Heart J. 2020;41:255-323.

[12] Haffner SM, Lehto S, Rönnemaa T, Pyörälä K, Laakso M. Mortality from coronary heart disease in subjects with type 2 diabetes and in nondiabetic subjects with and without prior myocardial infarction. N Engl J Med. 1998;339:229-34.

[13] Juutilainen A, Lehto S, Rönnemaa T, Pyörälä K, Laakso M. Type 2 diabetes as a "coronary heart disease equivalent": an 18-year prospective population-based study in Finnish subjects. Diabetes Care. 2005;28:2901-7.

[14] Vinik AI, Erbas T, Park TS, Nolan R, Pittenger GL. Platelet dysfunction in type 2 diabetes. Diabetes Care. 2001;24:1476-85.

[15] Ferroni P, Basili S, Falco A, Davì G. Platelet activation in type 2 diabetes mellitus. J Thromb Haemost. 2004;2:1282-91.

[16] Neumann F-J, Sousa-Uva M, Ahlsson A, Alfonso F, Banning AP, Benedetto U, et al. 2018 ESC/EACTS Guidelines on myocardial revascularization. Eur Heart J. 2019;40:87-165.

[17] Iakovou I, Schmidt T, Bonizzoni E, Ge L, Sangiorgi GM, Stankovic G, et al. Incidence, predictors, and outcome of thrombosis after successful implantation of drug-eluting stents. JAMA. 2005;293:2126-30.

[18] Angiolillo DJ. Antiplatelet therapy in type 2 diabetes mellitus. Curr Opin Endocrinol Diabetes Obes. 2007;14:124-31.

[19] Reaven GM. Banting lecture 1988. Role of insulin resistance in human disease. Diabetes. 1988;37:1595-607.

[20] Grant PJ. Diabetes mellitus as a prothrombotic condition. J Intern Med. 2007;262:157-72.

[21] O'Driscoll G, Green D, Rankin J, Stanton K, Taylor R. Improvement in endothelial function by angiotensin converting enzyme inhibition in insulin-dependent diabetes mellitus. J Clin Invest. 1997;100:678-84.

[22] Schmidt AM, Yan SD, Wautier JL, Stern D. Activation of receptor for advanced glycation end products: a mechanism for chronic vascular dysfunction in diabetic vasculopathy and atherosclerosis. Circ Res. 1999;84:489-97.

[23] Schmidt AM, Hori O, Brett J, Yan SD, Wautier JL, Stern D. Cellular receptors for advanced glycation end products. Implications for induction of oxidant stress and cellular dysfunction in the pathogenesis of vascular lesions. Arterioscler Thromb. 1994;14:1521-8.

[24] Dresner A, Laurent D, Marcucci M, Griffin ME, Dufour S, Cline GW, et al. Effects of free fatty acids on glucose transport and IRS-1-associated phosphatidylinositol 3-kinase activity. J Clin Invest. 1999;103:253-9.

[25] Dichtl W, Nilsson L, Goncalves I, Ares MP, Banfi C, Calara F, et al. Very low-density lipoprotein activates nuclear factor-kappaB in endothelial cells. Circ Res. 1999;84:1085-94.

[26] Inoguchi T, Li P, Umeda F, Yu HY, Kakimoto M, Imamura M, et al. High glucose level and free fatty acid stimulate reactive oxygen species production through protein kinase C--dependent activation of NAD(P)H oxidase in cultured vascular cells. Diabetes. 2000;49:1939-45.

[27] O'Neill WW. Multivessel balloon angioplasty should be abandoned in diabetic patients! J Am Coll Cardiol. 1998;31:20-2.

[28] Oliver FJ, de la Rubia G, Feener EP, Lee ME, Loeken MR, Shiba T, et al. Stimulation of endothelin-1 gene expression by insulin in endothelial cells. J Biol Chem. 1991;266:23251-6.

[29] Ferri C, Pittoni V, Piccoli A, Laurenti O, Cassone MR, Bellini C, et al. Insulin stimulates endothelin-1 secretion from human endothelial cells and modulates its circulating levels in vivo. J Clin Endocrinol Metab. 1995;80:829-35.

[30] Piatti PM, Monti LD, Conti M, Baruffaldi L, Galli L, Phan CV, et al. Hypertriglyceridemia and hyperinsulinemia are potent inducers of endothelin-1 release in humans. Diabetes. 1996;45:316-21.

[31] Wolpert HA, Steen SN, Istfan NW, Simonson DC. Insulin modulates circulating endothelin-1 levels in humans. Metab Clin Exp. 1993;42:1027-30.

[32] Stout RW. Insulin and atheroma. 20-yr perspective. Diabetes Care. 1990;13:631-54.

[33] Nishimoto Y, Miyazaki Y, Toki Y, Murakami R, Shinoda M, Fukushima A, et al. Enhanced secretion of insulin plays a role in the development of atherosclerosis and restenosis of coronary arteries: elective percutaneous transluminal coronary angioplasty in patients with effort angina. J Am Coll Cardiol. 1998;32:1624-9.

[34] Osanai H, Kanayama H, Miyazaki Y, Fukushima A, Shinoda M, Ito T. Usefulness of enhanced insulin secretion during an oral glucose tolerance test as a predictor of restenosis after direct percutaneous transluminal coronary angioplasty during acute myocardial infarction in patients without diabetes mellitus. Am J Cardiol. 1998;81:698-701.

[35] Takagi T, Yoshida K, Akasaka T, Kaji S, Kawamoto T, Honda Y, et al. Hyperinsulinemia during oral glucose tolerance test is associated with increased neointimal tissue proliferation after coronary stent implantation in nondiabetic patients: a serial intravascular ultrasound study. J Am Coll Cardiol. 2000;36:731-8.

[36] Baldi S, Natali A, Buzzigoli G, Galvan AQ, Sironi AM, Ferrannini E. In vivo effect of insulin on intracellular calcium concentrations: relation to insulin resistance. Metab Clin Exp. 1996;45:1402-7.

[37] Angiolillo DJ, Bernardo E, Sabaté M, Jimenez-Quevedo P, Costa MA, Palazuelos J, et al. Impact of platelet reactivity on cardiovascular outcomes in patients with type 2 diabetes mellitus and coronary artery disease. J Am Coll Cardiol. 2007;50:1541-7.

[38] Angiolillo DJ, Bernardo E, Ramírez C, Costa MA, Sabaté M, Jimenez-Quevedo P, et al. Insulin therapy is associated with platelet dysfunction in patients with type 2 diabetes mellitus on dual oral antiplatelet treatment. J Am Coll Cardiol. 2006;48:298-304.

[39] Davì G, Averna M, Catalano I, Barbagallo CM, Giovenco E, Carroccio A, et al. Platelet function in patients with type 2 diabetes mellitus: the effect of glycaemic control. Diabetes Res. 1989;10:7-12.

[40] Wallentin L, Varenhorst C, James S, Erlinge D, Braun OO, Jakubowski JA, et al. Prasugrel achieves greater and faster P2Y12receptor-mediated platelet inhibition than clopidogrel due to more efficient generation of its active metabolite in aspirin-treated patients with coronary artery disease. Eur Heart J. 2008;29:21-30.

[41] Wiviott SD, Braunwald E, McCabe CH, Montalescot G, Ruzyllo W, Gottlieb S, et al. Prasugrel versus clopidogrel in patients with acute coronary syndromes. N Engl J Med. 2007;357:2001-15.

[42] Wiviott SD, Braunwald E, Angiolillo DJ, Meisel S, Dalby AJ, Verheugt FWA, et al. Greater clinical benefit of more intensive oral antiplatelet therapy with prasugrel in patients with diabetes mellitus in the trial to assess improvement in therapeutic outcomes by optimizing platelet inhibition with prasugrel-Thrombolysis in Myocardial Infarction 38. Circulation. 2008;118:1626-36.

[43] Angiolillo DJ, Badimon JJ, Saucedo JF, Frelinger AL, Michelson AD, Jakubowski JA, et al. A pharmacodynamic comparison of prasugrel vs. high-dose clopidogrel in patients with type 2 diabetes mellitus and coronary artery disease: results of the Optimizing anti-Platelet Therapy In diabetes MellitUS (OPTIMUS)-3 Trial. Eur Heart J. 2011;32:838-46.

[44] Gurbel PA, Bliden KP, Butler K, Antonino MJ, Wei C, Teng R, et al. Response to ticagrelor in clopidogrel nonresponders and responders and effect of switching therapies: the RESPOND study. Circulation. 2010;121:1188-99.

[45] James S, Angiolillo DJ, Cornel JH, Erlinge D, Husted S, Kontny F, et al. Ticagrelor vs. clopidogrel in patients with acute coronary syndromes and diabetes: a substudy from the PLATelet inhibition and patient Outcomes (PLATO) trial. Eur Heart J. 2010;31:3006-16.

[46] Hindricks G, Potpara T, Dagres N, Arbelo E, Bax JJ, Blomström-Lundqvist C, et al. 2020 ESC Guidelines for the diagnosis and management of atrial fibrillation developed in collaboration with the European Association of Cardio-Thoracic Surgery (EACTS). Eur Heart J. 2020;

[47] Gibson WJ, Gibson CM, Yee MK, Korjian S, Daaboul Y, Plotnikov AN, et al. Safety and Efficacy of Rivaroxaban When Added to Aspirin Monotherapy Among Stabilized Post-Acute Coronary Syndrome Patients: A Pooled Analysis Study of ATLAS ACS-TIMI 46 and ATLAS ACS 2-TIMI 51. J Am Heart Assoc [Internet]. 2019 [cited 2020 Oct 4];8. Available from: https://www.ncbi.nlm.nih.gov/pmc/articles/PMC6474929/

[48] Eikelboom JW, Connolly SJ, Bosch J, Dagenais GR, Hart RG, Shestakovska O, et al. Rivaroxaban with or without Aspirin in Stable Cardiovascular Disease. N Engl J Med. 2017;377:1319-30.

[49] Rensing BJ, Hermans WR, Vos J, Tijssen JG, Rutch W, Danchin N, et al. Luminal narrowing after percutaneous transluminal coronary angioplasty. A study of clinical, procedural, and lesional factors related to long-term angiographic outcome. Coronary Artery Restenosis Prevention on Repeated Thromboxane Antagonism (CARPORT) Study Group. Circulation. 1993;88:975-85.

[50] Kimura T, Kaburagi S, Tamura T, Yokoi H, Nakagawa Y, Yokoi H, et al. Remodeling of human coronary arteries undergoing coronary angioplasty or atherectomy. Circulation. 1997;96:475-83.

[51] Mintz GS, Popma JJ, Pichard AD, Kent KM, Satler LF, Wong C, et al. Arterial remodeling after coronary angioplasty: a serial intravascular ultrasound study. Circulation. 1996;94:35-43.

[52] Garg P, Normand S-LT, Silbaugh TS, Wolf RE, Zelevinsky K, Lovett A, et al. Drug-eluting or bare-metal stenting in patients with diabetes mellitus: results from the Massachusetts Data Analysis Center Registry. Circulation. 2008;118:2277-85, 7p following 2285.

[53] Fischman DL, Leon MB, Baim DS, Schatz RA, Savage MP, Penn I, et al. A randomized comparison of coronary-stent placement and balloon angioplasty in the treatment of coronary artery disease. Stent Restenosis Study Investigators. N Engl J Med. 1994;331:496-501.

[54] Serruys PW, de Jaegere P, Kiemeneij F, Macaya C, Rutsch W, Heyndrickx G, et al. A comparison of balloon-expandable-stent implantation with balloon angioplasty in patients with coronary artery disease. Benestent Study Group. N Engl J Med. 1994;331:489-95.

[55] Van Belle E, Périé M, Braune D, Chmaït A, Meurice T, Abolmaali K, et al. effects of coronary stenting on vessel patency and long-term clinical outcome after percutaneous coronary revascularization in diabetic patients. Journal of the American College of Cardiology. 2002;40:410-7.

[56] West Nick E.J., Ruygrok Peter N., Disco Clemens M.C., Webster Mark W.I., Lindeboom Wietze K., O'Neill William W., et al. Clinical and Angiographic Predictors of Restenosis After Stent Deployment in Diabetic Patients. Circulation. 2004;109:867-73.

[57] Takagi T, Akasaka T, Yamamuro A, Honda Y, Hozumi T, Morioka S, et al. Troglitazone reduces neointimal tissue proliferation after coronary stent implantation in patients with non-insulin dependent diabetes mellitus: a serial intravascular ultrasound study. J Am Coll Cardiol. 2000;36:1529-35.

[58] Weber FD, Schneider H, Wiemer M, Pfannebecker T, Tebbe U, Hamm CW, et al. Sirolimus eluting stent (Cypher) in patients with diabetes mellitus: results from the German Cypher Stent Registry. Clin Res Cardiol. 2008;97:105-9.

[59] Hermiller JB, Raizner A, Cannon L, Gurbel PA, Kutcher MA, Wong SC, et al. Outcomes with the polymer-based paclitaxel-eluting TAXUS stent in patients with diabetes mellitus: the TAXUS-IV trial. J Am Coll Cardiol. 2005;45:1172-9.

[60] Moses JW, Leon MB, Popma JJ, Fitzgerald PJ, Holmes DR, O'Shaughnessy C, et al. Sirolimus-eluting stents versus standard stents in patients with stenosis in a native coronary artery. N Engl J Med. 2003;349:1315-23.

[61] Moussa I, Leon MB, Baim DS, O'Neill WW, Popma JJ, Buchbinder M, et al. Impact of sirolimus-eluting stents on outcome in diabetic patients: a SIRIUS (SIRolImUS-coated Bx Velocity balloon-expandable stent in the treatment of patients with de novo coronary artery lesions) substudy. Circulation. 2004;109:2273-8.

[62] Ellis SG, Stone GW, Cox DA, Hermiller J, O'Shaughnessy C, Mann T, et al. Long-term safety and efficacy with paclitaxel-eluting stents: 5-year final results of the TAXUS IV clinical trial (TAXUS IV-SR: Treatment of De Novo Coronary Disease Using a Single Paclitaxel-Eluting Stent). JACC Cardiovasc Interv. 2009;2:1248-59.

[63] Sabaté M, Jiménez-Quevedo P, Angiolillo DJ, Gómez-Hospital JA, Alfonso F, Hernández-Antolín R, et al. Randomized comparison of sirolimus-eluting stent versus standard stent for percutaneous coronary revascularization in diabetic patients: the diabetes and sirolimus-eluting stent (DIABETES) trial. Circulation. 2005;112:2175-83.

[64] Jiménez-Quevedo P, Hernando L, Gómez-Hospital JA, Iñiguez A, SanRoman A, Alfonso F, et al. Sirolimus-eluting stent versus bare metal stent in diabetic patients: the final five-year follow-up of the DIABETES trial. EuroIntervention. 2013;9:328-35.

[65] One-year results of the SCORPIUS study: a German multicenter investigation on the effectiveness of sirolimus-eluting stents in diabetic patients | Cochrane Library [Internet]. [cited 2020 Sep 18]. Available from: https://www.cochranelibrary.com/es/central/doi/10.1002/central/CN-00705649/related-content

[66] Sinning J-M, Baumgart D, Werner N, Klauss V, Baer FM, Hartmann F, et al. Five-year results of the Multicenter Randomized Controlled Open-Label Study of the CYPHER Sirolimus-Eluting Stent in the Treatment of Diabetic Patients with De Novo Native Coronary Artery Lesions (SCORPIUS) study: a German multicenter investigation on the effectiveness of sirolimus-eluting stents in diabetic patients. Am Heart J. 2012;163:446-53, 453.e1.

[67] Maresta A, Varani E, Balducelli M, Varbella F, Lettieri C, Uguccioni L, et al. Comparison of effectiveness and safety

of sirolimus-eluting stents versus bare-metal stents in patients with diabetes mellitus (from the Italian Multicenter Randomized DESSERT Study). Am J Cardiol. 2008;101:1560-6.

[68] Chan C, Zambahari R, Kaul U, Lau CP, Whitworth H, Cohen S, et al. A randomized comparison of sirolimus-eluting versus bare metal stents in the treatment of diabetic patients with native coronary artery lesions: The DECODE study. Catheterization and Cardiovascular Interventions. 2008;72:591-600.

[69] Stettler C, Allemann S, Wandel S, Kastrati A, Morice MC, Schömig A, et al. Drug eluting and bare metal stents in people with and without diabetes: collaborative network meta-analysis. BMJ. 2008;337:a1331.

[70] Windecker S, Remondino A, Eberli FR, Jüni P, Räber L, Wenaweser P, et al. Sirolimus-eluting and paclitaxel-eluting stents for coronary revascularization. N Engl J Med. 2005;353:653-62.

[71] Dibra A, Kastrati A, Mehilli J, Pache J, Schühlen H, von Beckerath N, et al. Paclitaxel-eluting or sirolimus-eluting stents to prevent restenosis in diabetic patients. N Engl J Med. 2005;353:663-70.

[72] Stone GW, Rizvi A, Sudhir K, Newman W, Applegate RJ, Cannon LA, et al. Randomized comparison of everolimus- and paclitaxel-eluting stents. 2-year follow-up from the SPIRIT (Clinical Evaluation of the XIENCE V Everolimus Eluting Coronary Stent System) IV trial. J Am Coll Cardiol. 2011;58:19-25.

[73] Grube E, Chevalier B, Guagliumi G, Smits PC, Stuteville M, Dorange C, et al. The SPIRIT V diabetic study: a randomized clinical evaluation of the XIENCE V everolimus-eluting stent vs the TAXUS Liberté paclitaxel-eluting stent in diabetic patients with de novo coronary artery lesions. Am Heart J. 2012;163:867-875.e1.

[74] Leon MB, Mauri L, Popma JJ, Cutlip DE, Nikolsky E, O'Shaughnessy C, et al. A randomized comparison of the Endeavor zotarolimus-eluting stent versus the TAXUS paclitaxel-eluting stent in de novo native coronary lesions 12-month outcomes from the ENDEAVOR IV trial. J Am Coll Cardiol. 2010;55:543-54.

[75] Serruys PW, Silber S, Garg S, van Geuns RJ, Richardt G, Buszman PE, et al. Comparison of zotarolimus-eluting and everolimus-eluting coronary stents. N Engl J Med. 2010;363:136-46.

[76] Wykrzykowska JJ, Räber L, de Vries T, Bressers M, Buszman P, Linke A, et al. Biolimus-eluting biodegradable polymer versus sirolimus-eluting permanent polymer stent performance in long lesions: results from the LEADERS multicentre trial substudy. EuroIntervention. 2009;5:310-7.

[77] Fröbert O, Lagerqvist B, Carlsson J, Lindbäck J, Stenestrand U, James SK. Differences in restenosis rate with different drug-eluting stents in patients with and without diabetes mellitus: a report from the SCAAR (Swedish Angiography and Angioplasty Registry). J Am Coll Cardiol. 2009;53:1660-7.

[78] Urban P, Gershlick AH, Guagliumi G, Guyon P, Lotan C, Schofer J, et al. Safety of coronary sirolimus-eluting stents in daily clinical practice: one-year follow-up of the e-Cypher registry. Circulation. 2006;113:1434-41.

[79] Stenestrand U, James SK, Lindbäck J, Fröbert O, Carlsson J, Scherstén F, et al. Safety and efficacy of drug-eluting vs. bare metal stents in patients with diabetes mellitus: long-term follow-up in the Swedish Coronary

Angiography and Angioplasty Registry (SCAAR). Eur Heart J. 2010;31:177-86.

[80] de Waha A, Dibra A, Kufner S, Baumgart D, Sabate M, Maresta A, et al. Long-term outcome after sirolimus-eluting stents versus bare metal stents in patients with diabetes mellitus: a patient-level meta-analysis of randomized trials. Clin Res Cardiol. 2011;100:561-70.

[81] Silber S, Windecker S, Vranckx P, Serruys PW. Unrestricted randomised use of two new generation drug-eluting coronary stents: 2-year patient-related versus stent-related outcomes from the RESOLUTE All Comers trial. The Lancet. 2011;377:1241-7.

[82] Rydén L, Standl E, Bartnik M, Van den Berghe G, Betteridge J, de Boer M-J, et al. Guidelines on diabetes, pre-diabetes, and cardiovascular diseases: executive summary. The Task Force on Diabetes and Cardiovascular Diseases of the European Society of Cardiology (ESC) and of the European Association for the Study of Diabetes (EASD). Eur Heart J. 2007;28:88-136.

[83] King SB, Kosinski AS, Guyton RA, Lembo NJ, Weintraub WS. Eight-year mortality in the Emory Angioplasty versus Surgery Trial (EAST). J Am Coll Cardiol. 2000;35:1116-21.

[84] BARI Investigators. The final 10-year follow-up results from the BARI randomized trial. J Am Coll Cardiol. 2007;49:1600-6.

[85] Henderson RA, Pocock SJ, Sharp SJ, Nanchahal K, Sculpher MJ, Buxton MJ, et al. Long-term results of RITA-1 trial: clinical and cost comparisons of coronary angioplasty and coronary-artery bypass grafting. Randomised Intervention Treatment of Angina. Lancet. 1998;352:1419-25.

[86] Kurbaan AS, Bowker TJ, Ilsley CD, Sigwart U, Rickards AF, CABRI Investigators (Coronary Angioplasty versus Bypass Revascularization Investigation). Difference in the mortality of the CABRI diabetic and nondiabetic populations and its relation to coronary artery disease and the revascularization mode. Am J Cardiol. 2001;87:947-50; A3.

[87] Abizaid A, Costa MA, Centemero M, Abizaid AS, Legrand VM, Limet RV, et al. Clinical and economic impact of diabetes mellitus on percutaneous and surgical treatment of multivessel coronary disease patients: insights from the Arterial Revascularization Therapy Study (ARTS) trial. Circulation. 2001;104:533-8.

[88] Sedlis SP, Morrison DA, Lorin JD, Esposito R, Sethi G, Sacks J, et al. Percutaneous coronary intervention versus coronary bypass graft surgery for diabetic patients with unstable angina and risk factors for adverse outcomes with bypass: Outcome of diabetic patients in the AWESOME randomized trial and registry. Journal of the American College of Cardiology. 2002;40:1555-66.

[89] Hlatky MA, Boothroyd DB, Bravata DM, Boersma E, Booth J, Brooks MM, et al. Coronary artery bypass surgery compared with percutaneous coronary interventions for multivessel disease: a collaborative analysis of individual patient data from ten randomised trials. Lancet. 2009;373:1190-7.

[90] Onuma Y, Wykrzykowska JJ, Garg S, Vranckx P, Serruys PW, ARTS I and II Investigators. 5-Year follow-up of coronary revascularization in diabetic patients with multivessel coronary artery disease: insights from ARTS (arterial revascularization therapy study)-II and ARTS-I trials. JACC Cardiovasc Interv. 2011;4:317-23.

[91] Rodriguez AE, Maree AO, Mieres J, Berrocal D, Grinfeld L,

Fernandez-Pereira C, et al. Late loss of early benefit from drug-eluting stents when compared with bare-metal stents and coronary artery bypass surgery: 3 years follow-up of the ERACI III registry. Eur Heart J. 2007;28:2118-25.

[92] Briguori C, Condorelli G, Airoldi F, Focaccio A, D'Andrea D, Cannavale M, et al. Comparison of coronary drug-eluting stents versus coronary artery bypass grafting in patients with diabetes mellitus. Am J Cardiol. 2007;99:779-84.

[93] Hannan EL, Wu C, Walford G, Culliford AT, Gold JP, Smith CR, et al. Drug-Eluting Stents vs. Coronary-Artery Bypass Grafting in Multivessel Coronary Disease. New England Journal of Medicine. 2008;358:331-41.

[94] Kappetein AP, Head SJ, Morice M-C, Banning AP, Serruys PW, Mohr F-W, et al. Treatment of complex coronary artery disease in patients with diabetes: 5-year results comparing outcomes of bypass surgery and percutaneous coronary intervention in the SYNTAX trial. Eur J Cardiothorac Surg. 2013;43:1006-13.

[95] Kapur A, Hall RJ, Malik IS, Qureshi AC, Butts J, de Belder M, et al. Randomized comparison of percutaneous coronary intervention with coronary artery bypass grafting in diabetic patients. 1-year results of the CARDia (Coronary Artery Revascularization in Diabetes) trial. J Am Coll Cardiol. 2010;55:432-40.

[96] Dangas GD, Farkouh ME, Sleeper LA, Yang M, Schoos MM, Macaya C, et al. Long-term outcome of PCI versus CABG in insulin and non-insulin-treated diabetic patients: results from the FREEDOM trial. J Am Coll Cardiol. 2014;64:1189-97.

[97] BARI 2D Study Group, Frye RL, August P, Brooks MM, Hardison RM, Kelsey SF, et al. A randomized trial of therapies for type 2 diabetes and coronary artery disease. N Engl J Med. 2009;360:2503-15.

[98] Head SJ, Milojevic M, Daemen J, Ahn J-M, Boersma E, Christiansen EH, et al. Mortality after coronary artery bypass grafting versus percutaneous coronary intervention with stenting for coronary artery disease: a pooled analysis of individual patient data. Lancet. 2018;391:939-48.

[99] Bavishi C, Baber U, Panwar S, Pirrotta S, Dangas GD, Moreno P, et al. Efficacy and safety of everolimus and zotarolimus-eluting stents versus first-generation drug-eluting stents in patients with diabetes: A meta-analysis of randomized trials. Int J Cardiol. 2017;230:310-8.

[100] Park S-J, Ahn J-M, Kim Y-H, Park D-W, Yun S-C, Lee J-Y, et al. Trial of everolimus-eluting stents or bypass surgery for coronary disease. N Engl J Med. 2015;372:1204-12.

[101] Stone GW, Sabik JF, Serruys PW, Simonton CA, Généreux P, Puskas J, et al. Everolimus-Eluting Stents or Bypass Surgery for Left Main Coronary Artery Disease. N Engl J Med. 2016;375:2223-35.

[102] Cutlip DE, Chhabra AG, Baim DS, Chauhan MS, Marulkar S, Massaro J, et al. Beyond restenosis: five-year clinical outcomes from second-generation coronary stent trials. Circulation. 2004;110:1226-30.

[103] Zellweger MJ, Kaiser C, Jeger R, Brunner-La Rocca H-P, Buser P, Bader F, et al. Coronary artery disease progression late after successful stent implantation. J Am Coll Cardiol. 2012;59:793-9.

[104] Weisz G, Leon MB, Holmes DR, Kereiakes DJ, Popma JJ, Teirstein PS, et al. Five-year follow-up after sirolimus-eluting stent implantation results of the SIRIUS (Sirolimus-Eluting

Stent in De-Novo Native Coronary Lesions) Trial. J Am Coll Cardiol. 2009;53:1488-97.

[105] Ellis SG, Stone GW, Cox DA, Hermiller J, O'Shaughnessy C, Mann T, et al. Long-term safety and efficacy with paclitaxel-eluting stents: 5-year final results of the TAXUS IV clinical trial (TAXUS IV-SR: Treatment of De Novo Coronary Disease Using a Single Paclitaxel-Eluting Stent). JACC Cardiovasc Interv. 2009;2:1248-59.

[106] Rozenman Y, Sapoznikov D, Mosseri M, Gilon D, Lotan C, Nassar H, et al. Long-term angiographic follow-up of coronary balloon angioplasty in patients with diabetes mellitus: a clue to the explanation of the results of the BARI study. Balloon Angioplasty Revascularization Investigation. J Am Coll Cardiol. 1997;30:1420-5.

[107] Kroncke GM, Kosolcharoen P, Clayman JA, Peduzzi PN, Detre K, Takaro T. Five-year changes in coronary arteries of medical and surgical patients of the Veterans Administration Randomized Study of Bypass Surgery. Circulation. 1988;78:I144-150.

Chapter 3

Radial Artery Access

Carmelo Panetta and Johnny Chahine

Abstract

Radial artery access for angiography has matured over the past two decades and is now the preferred point of access for most patients. Lower bleeding rates in clinical randomized trials have translated into lower mortality prompting change in the guidelines. Advances in technique with use of ultrasound for access to properly size the sheath, proper dosing of anticoagulation and new techniques for sheath removal have dramatically lowered radial artery occlusion rates. Radial artery spasm has improved with vasodilators and proper sedation. Advances in support boards and sheath extension have opened up left radial access. Advances in lower profile sheaths and sheathless systems allow larger catheters in smaller arteries. Advances in longer balloons and sheaths have opened up radial access for peripheral interventions. Areas of clinical research include use of ulnar artery compared to radial, left versus right radial access, use of radial artery for a surgical conduit after angiography, radiation exposure and advantage of radial approach in the elderly.

Keywords: radial artery, ulnar artery, radial artery occlusion, sheathless guide, left radial support

1. Introduction

Radial artery access for angiography was first described in 1948 via cut down and direct insertion into either right or left radial artery [1], and in 1989 direct coronary angiography with percutaneous access via left radial artery [2]. Since then, radial artery access has advanced catheterization for patients by reducing vascular site bleeding which translated into both lower mortality and lower costs [3, 4]. Lesser known advantages include opening up both femoral arteries for larger sheaths for both hemodynamic support, complex coronary, peripheral or structural cases, as well as patient satisfaction. Acceptance has been slow by operators given the artery is smaller, orthopedic concerns of the operator with left radial and navigating catheters thru tortuous vascular anatomy, resulting in longer cases and higher radiation exposure [5, 6]. Advances in both techniques and medical devices have overcome many of the concerns opening up the wrist arteries for a far greater number than the past, translating into benefits for patients, hospitals and physicians.

2. Outline for the chapter

1. Bleeding reduction and impact on mortality

2. Ultrasound access

3. RAO: prevention/therapy

4. Radial Access Support

5. Thin walled sheaths and Sheathless guides

6. Peripheral interventions via radial approach

7. Areas of research: ulnar vs. radial; use of radial for graft; radiation exposure; elderly

3. Bleeding reduction and impact on mortality

Radial access found a niche initially by patient preference and potential benefit given the complications with femoral or brachial access [1]. Radial artery access for coronary angiography and percutaneous intervention is deemed safer than femoral access, positively impacting mortality, and bleeding risk.

A multicenter randomized controlled trial involving 8404 participants with acute coronary syndrome found that using radial access decreases major bleeding [RR 0.67 (0.49–0.92), $p = 0.01$] and all-cause mortality [RR 0.72 (0.53–0.99), $p = 0.045$] compared to femoral access [7]. The RIFLE-STECAS trial involved only patients with ST-elevation myocardial infarction (STEMI) ($n = 1001$), and found lower bleeding rates (7.8% vs. 12.2%, $p = 0.026$) and cardiac mortality in the radial access group (5.2% vs. 9.2%, $p = 0.02$), and decreased median length of stay [5 [4–7] days vs. 6 [5–8], $p = 0.03$] [8]. The RIVAL trial separately studied the outcomes of STEMI ($n = 1958$) and non-ST elevation acute coronary syndrome ($n = 5063$) patients. Survival benefit and decreased bleeding risk with radial access was seen in the STEMI group [9]. A comparative study of STEMI patients in cardiogenic shock after PCI ($n = 2663$) showed that 1-year mortality was lower using the transradial approach compared to transfemoral (44% vs. 64%, $p = 0.004$), with radial artery access being an independent predictor of 1-year mortality [HR 0.65 (0.42–0.98), $p = 0.041$] [10]. The rate of TIMI 3 flow was identical in both groups. Major bleeding was higher in the femoral group (25% vs. 13%, $p = 0.04$) as well as bleeding related to access site (9 vs. 0.9%, $p = 0.01$) [10]. The STEMI-RADIAL trial also involved STEMI patients ($n = 707$), and found decreased composite endpoint of death, myocardial infarction, stroke, major bleeding, and vascular complications (4.6% vs. 11%, $p = 0.003$) but similar mortality rates at 30 days (2.3% vs. 3.1%, $p = 0.64$) and 6 months (2.3% vs. 3.6%, $p = 0.31$) [11]. The SAFARI-STEMI trial enrolled 2292 out of 4800 patients, halted prematurely because of futility finding 30-day mortality was similar between the radial and femoral access groups (RR 1.15 (0.58–2.30), $p = 0.69$). There was no difference in bleeding risk [RR 0.71 (0.38–1.33), $p = 0.28$] [12]. These findings can be explained by the fact that the proceduralists were experienced cardiologists at high-volume centers, a closure device was used in 68% of patients in the femoral group, less 2b3a inhibitor was used and bivalirudin was favored in 92% of those patients, which is known to cause less bleeding than heparin [12].

Yet the totality of data from 12 randomized clinical trials over the past decade found particularly in those with acute coronary syndrome, a lower bleeding rate translated into lower mortality [3]. This prompted a radial first approach by the American Heart Association for those with acute coronary syndrome [3].

4. Ultrasound access

Ultrasound (US) for radial access from several smaller studies implied a benefit in time to access [13, 14]. The RAUST trial included 698 patients and showed that an ultrasound-guided approach decreased the number of attempts (mean 1.65 ± 1.2 vs. 3.05 3.4, p < 0.0001) and the time to getting access (88 ± 78 seconds vs. 108 ± 112 seconds, p = 0.006) [15]. In another randomized controlled trial performed in Australia that enrolled 1388 patients, ultrasound use decreased time to getting access (93 vs. 11 seconds, p = 0.009), the number of attempts (1.47 vs. 1.9, p < 0.0001) with increased chances of success from the first try (73% vs. 59.7%, p < 0.0001) [16]. Besides the faster and higher success rate, pre-puncture ultrasound can prevent vascular complications by properly sizing the radial artery to sheath diameter [17].

5. RAO: prevention/therapy

Radial artery occlusion (RAO) is common and is seen in up to 10% of patients early after the procedure, although the more recent trials (after 2018) showed an RAO rate of less than 3.7% [18].

Multiple preventive techniques have been described including importance of anticoagulation, proper sizing of the radial artery to sheath/guide, patent hemostasis, prophylactic ulnar compression and shorten duration of compression [18]. A meta-analysis that included 31,345 patients and 66 studies concluded that high dose heparin (5000 IU) administration decreased the risk of RAO by 64%, and reducing compression times decreased this risk by 72% [19]. A recent study of high dose (100 IU/kg body weight) versus (50 IU/kg/body weight) lowered RAO [20]. That is why it has been recommended to administer at 5000 U or 50 or higher IU/kg body weight unfractionated heparin for all procedures with radial artery access [18, 21]. Importance of having sheath to radial artery diameter < 1.0 is considered best for reducing RAO [18, 21], pushing industry to provide sheaths with thinner walls or sheathless guide systems. The 6.5 F sheathless Eaucath appeared to have lower RAO compared to thin walled 6F sheath, 0.0% vs. 2.0%, p 0.031 with sample size of 600 randomized patients [22]. Although thinner, the RAP and BEAT (Radial Artery Patency and Bleeding, Efficacy, Adverse evenT) trial found thin walled 6French (F) sheath failed noninferiority to 5F sheath, (3.7% vs. 1.7%, pnon-inferiority = 0.150) [23]. Even a difference of 0.24 mm (5F standard with 2.22 mm vs. thin-walled 6F with 2.44 mm) may have lower RAO, implying smaller is better. Reduction of RAO rates have been reported after subcutaneous injection of nitroglycerin at the radial access site before the procedure (5% vs. 14%, P = 0.04) and the use of intraarterial nitroglycerin after the procedure (8% vs. 12%, p = 0.006) [24]. Maintaining radial artery patency during hemostasis is proven to reduce RAO rates, or patent hemostasis [18, 21]. This can be achieved by periodically monitoring oximetry-plethysmography after the procedure to ensure radial flow [25] Pneumatic radial compression based on the patient's mean arterial pressure and concomitant ulnar compression to increase radial flow have also been shown to be beneficial [26].

6. Radial access support

Support for access in the wrist has advanced over the past decade, with a focus on left arm support, radiation protection and having a board to hold equipment.

There has been a surge in the last several years to use the left wrist to circumvent challenges with access to the left internal mammary artery post coronary artery bypass surgery (CABG), those older than 75 years, short statue less than 5 foot five inches (1.65meters), and long term hypertension [5, 27]. Wrist access requires support for: access in the artery, management of equipment, radiation exposure along with comfort of the patient and the operator. Right arm support has advanced with arm extension boards to help with access, for example Radial Runway (TZ Medical), Rad Rest (Merit) or STAR system (Adept Medical) to help with access of the artery, especially useful if not using ultrasound **(Figure 1)**. Right boards include the Cardiotrap (Radial Solutions) (**Figure 2a**), EGGNEST from EGG medical (**Figure 2b**), STARSYSTEM by Adept Medical, Rad Board from Merit provides both arm support and radiation protection. The left arm support for both access and arm support across the abdomen is the Left Arm Support System by LP Medical **(Figure 2c)** and Cardiotrap from Radial Solutions. Other options for arm support alone include STARSYSTEM by Adept Medical, Cobra Board by TZ medical (**Figure 2d**), left radial support sling by Academic Health Science Network and Tesslagra sterile sleeve by Tesslagra Design Solutions. Once access is made for the left wrist and arm is placed across the abdomen, use of sheath extension such as the StandTall by

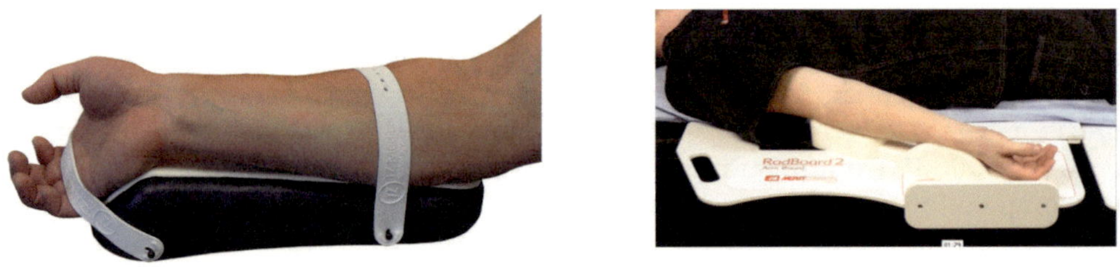

(a) (b)

Figure 1.
Devices to hold the wrist out to assist in accessing the radial artery. a. Radial Runway©, TZ medical. b. Rad Board© and Rad Rest©, Merit Medical.

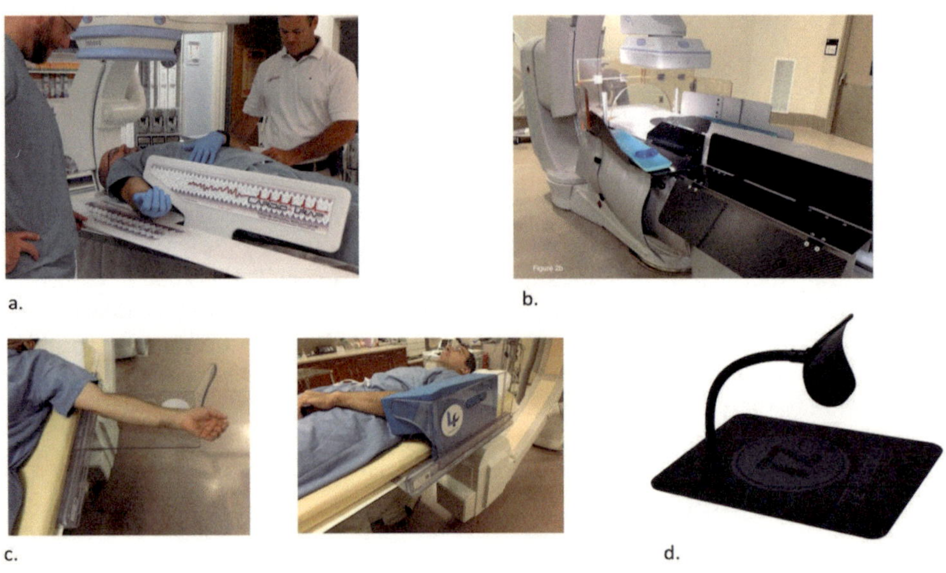

Figure 2.
Arm support systems. Right arm: a. Cardiotrap® (Transradial solutions, SC) b. EGG Nest® (EGG Medical, MN) c. Left arm support system (LASS) (LP Medical, MN) d. Cobra Board® (TZ Medical, OR).

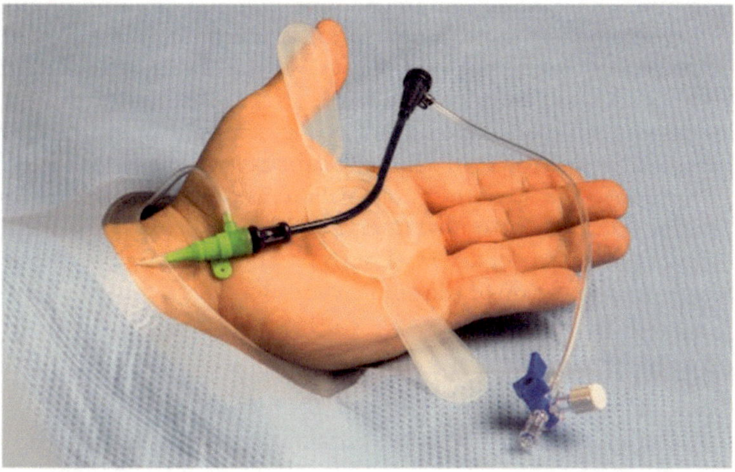

Figure 3.
Sheath Extension Standtall® (Radux Devices, MN).

Radux (**Figure 3**), distal radial approach or having a long sheath partly extended out (although risk for kinking of the sheath) will allow the physician to have an upright position on the right side of the patient while manipulating the catheter or guide.

7. Thin walled sheaths and Sheathless guides

Small diameter of the radial or ulnar artery has been overcome with thinner sheaths. For example the Slender (Terumo) (**Figure 4**) 6F outer diameter is 2.46 mm versus 2.62 mm for standard sheath outer diameter and the Slender 7F drops the outer diameter from 2.95 down to 2.79 mm. The downside is kinking of the thinner walled sheaths especially if partly inserted into the artery.

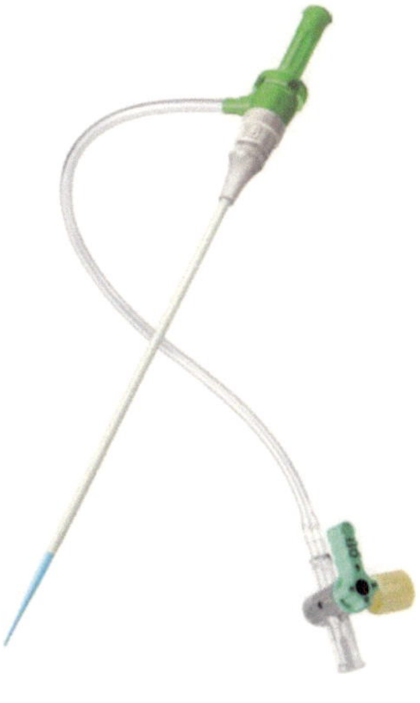

Figure 4.
Thin walled sheath, GLIDESHEATH SLENDER® Introducer Sheath – ©2020 Terumo Medical Corporation. All rights reserved.

Sheathless guides (Eaucath system from Asahi Intecc Co Ltd. or Railway system from Cordis) have opened up radial access for smaller arteries. The OD of the 6.5Fr SheathLess Eaucath is 2.16 mm, similar to the OD of the 4Fr sheath at 2.00 mm. The OD of the 7.5Fr SheathLess Eaucath is 2.49 mm, similar to the OD of the 5Fr sheath at 2.29 mm. The passing of the sheathless guide requires special attention to withdrawing the dilator before entry into the aorta from the subclavian. One other option is the use of an inflated balloon in the tip of the guide prior to passing into the artery referred to balloon-assisted shealthless transradial intervention (BASTI) [28]. The challenge is the use of 0.014 wire for support versus 0.021 or 0.035 and, as with sheathless guides one other issue is over manipulation of the guide without a sheath could induce spasm.

8. Peripheral interventions via radial approach

Peripheral interventions have adopted radial access to lower bleeding or due to hostile femoral artery anatomy [29]. Peripheral interventions include aorta, visceral, iliac/femoral and, rarely, popliteal [29, 30]. The learning curve for radial approach for peripheral interventions [29] may account for an increase in radiation [31]. Distance from the wrist to the site of percutaneous intervention is a limitation. Longer sheaths such as destination sheath by Terumo (**Figure 5a)** have allowed improved positioning for equipment. As with the sheathless guide, careful attention should be placed on pulling back the dilator before entering the aorta. Longer catheters have been developed by Terumo under the radial to peripheral program, (R2P) with shafts upto 200 cm including both balloons and self expanding peripheral stents (**Figure 5b).** Other companies have 170 cm catheter lengths including: Ultraverse RX (Bard); the Advance 14LP low Profile balloon (Cook); and the Armada 14 (Abbott), Mini Ghost (B.Braun), Steriling SL Monorail (Boston Scientific), Sleep OTW (Cordis) and Amphirion Deep OTW (Medtronic) all with catheters upto 150 cm in length. The longer shafts have furthered the use of radial access, along with left arm support and sheath extension but limited length of catheters with covered stents or drug coated balloons for infrainguinal disease [32].

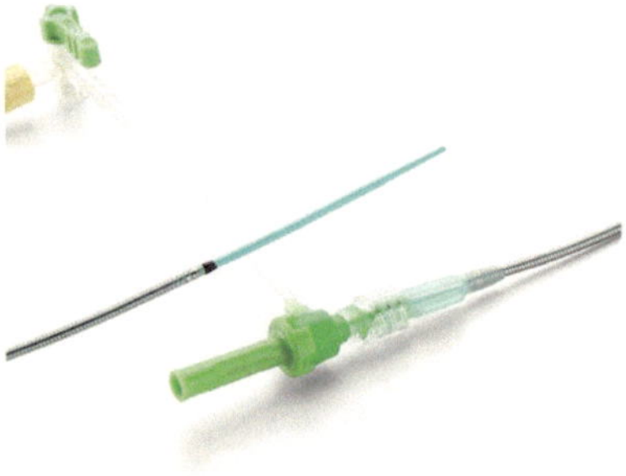

a.

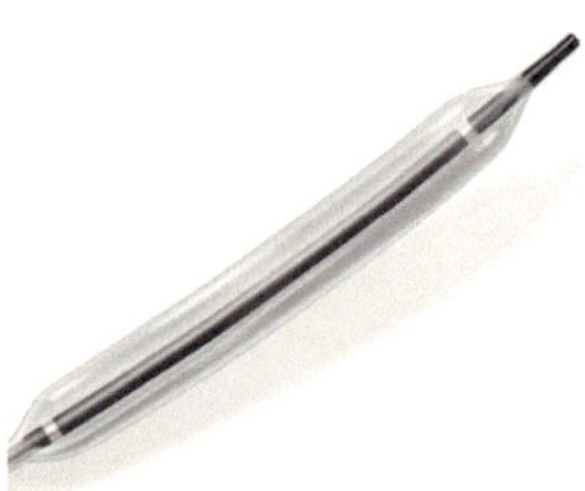

b.

Figure 5.
Long sheath R2PTM DESTINATION SLENDERTM Guiding Sheath b. 200 cm Long shaft R2PTM METACROSS® RX PTA Balloon Dilatation Catheter - ©2020 Terumo Medical Corporation. All rights reserved.

9. Areas of research

With an increase in clinical studies showing the advantages of radial access also came insight into complications including radial loops, high take off of radial artery, spasm, dissection [5]. The ulnar artery became another option, initially avoided due to location, as the ulnar artery is often deeper beneath the skin and concern for ulnar nerve damage or hand ischemia but reports for both coronary and peripheral angiography and interventions rasie doubts regarding those concerns [33–35]. A meta analysis of five trials found similar complications between radial vs. ulnar approach [36]., crossover was higher with ulnar versus radial approach but this was driven by one trial [37]. This trial was to enroll 2286 patients but was stopped early with 902 enrolled after finding cross over to another site was 26% more likely with ulnar approach compared to radial, with the caveat that ultrasound was not used for access. Further studies are warranted in comparing radial versus ulnar using ultrasound.

Radial artery is being reinvestigated as a favored coronary artery bypass graft (CABG) over veins with recent meta analysis of 1036 patients having lower mortality with arterial grafts over venous grafts [38]. This has prompted the ROMA prospective randomized trial comparing vein to arterial grafts for CABG. One study from 2003 found radial grafts that were previously cannulated had a lower patency rate [39]. Several other studies have found changes in the radial artery including arterial tears, radial intimal hyperplasia and loss of reactivity after sheath insertion [40–42]. This has prompted some surgeons to request interventional cardiologists not to use nondominant radial artery for angiography. Further studies investigating radial or ulnar access prior to CABG are recommended.

Radiation exposure is a constant worry in the catheterization laboratory [43]. Advances in technology have lowered radiation exposure including improved shielding. Clinical data have shown radial, particularly right radial, to have more radiation exposure compared to femoral approach [6]. Comparison of left radial to femoral approach in one randomized trial [44] found higher radiation compared in radial approach, although this was done prior to newer technology to assist in left radial such as sheath extension (eg. Stand Tall, Radux Devices) and left arm support systems. Multiple randomized trials found less radiation with left versus right radial [45–49] although one trial found more radiation with left radial [50]. Avoiding steep angles, particularly LAO -Caudal, lower magnification, lower frame rate with fluoroscopy, and distance is recommended [51, 52]. Further research comparing access sites is warranted to better understand with current technology the risks of radiation exposure.

Elderly have higher risk for CV procedures [53, 54] and benefits of radial approach for reduction in bleeding complications is a valid concern. Age appears to be a predictor of failure or cross over to another site [5, 19]. Yet studies in the elderly including a retrospective analysis have not shown increased time to treat ST elevation myocardial infarction [55]. A review of patients enrolled in randomized Rival trial found less complications but higher cross over rates in the elderly [56]. Further studies are warranted in those 75 years and older to compare radial (left versus right) and femoral access points in examining cross over rates, radiation, bleeding and success.

Radial access has dramatically changed over the past twenty years with advances in both technology and technique to bring this approach to the forefront in both the acute setting as well as for complex procedures.

Conflict of interest

Carmelo Panetta is co-owner of LP Medical LLC. Johnny Chahine has no conflict of interest.

Author details

Carmelo Panetta* and Johnny Chahine
University of Minnesota, Minneapolis, USA

*Address all correspondence to: panet002@umn.edu

References

[1] Radner S. 1948. "Thoracal aortaography by catheterization from the radial artery; preliminary report of a new technique." *Acta radiol* 29 (2): 178-80.

[2] Campeau L 1989. "Percutaneous Radial Artery Approach for Coroanry Angiography." *Catheter Cardiovasc Interv* 16: 3-7.

[3] Mason PJ, Shah B, Tamis-Holland JE et al. 2018. "An Update on Radial Artery Access and Best Practices for Transradial Coronary Angiography and Intervention in Acute Coronary elevation." *Circ Cardiovasc interv* 2018 Sept; 11(9):e000035.

[4] Mitchell MD, Hong JA, Lee BY et al. 2012. "Systematic Review and Cost-Benefit Analysis of Radial Artery Access for Coronary Angiography and Intervention." *Circ Cardiovasc Qual Outcomes* 5: 454-62.

[5] Dehghani P et al. 2009. "Mechanism and predictors of failed trasnradial approach for percutaneous coronary interventions." *J Am Coll Cardiol Intv* 2: 1057-64.

[6] Sciahbasi A, Frigoli E, Sarandrea A et al. 2017. "Radiation Exposure and Vascular Accss in Acute Coronary Syndromes: The RAD-Matrix Trial." *J Am Coll Cardiol.* 69 (20): 2530-37.

[7] Valgimigli M, Gagnor A, Calabro P et al. 2015. "Radial versus femoral access in patients with acute coronary syndromes undergoing invasive management: A randomized multicentre trial." *Lancet* 385 (9986): 2465-76.

[8] Romagnoli E, Biondi-Zoccai G, Sciahbasi A et al. 2012. "Radial versus femoral randomized investigation in ST-segment elevation acute coronary syndrome. The RIFLE-STEACS (radial versus femoral randomzied intrvesitatein ST_elevation Acute coronary syndrome) study." *J Am Coll Cardiol* 60 (24): 2481-89.

[9] Mehta ST, Joll SS, Claimes J, et al. 2012. "RIVAL Investitagors. Effects ofradial versus femoral artery access in patients iwth acute coronary syndrome with or without ST-Segment elevation." *J Am Coll Cardiol* 60: 2490-99

[10] Bernat I, Abdelaal E, Plourde G, Bataille Y, Cech J, Pesek J, et al. Early and late outcomes after primary percutaneous coronary intervention by radial or femoral approach in patients presenting in acute ST-elevation myocardial infarction and cardiogenic shock. Am Heart J [Internet]. 2013 Mar [cited 2020 Sep 22];165(3):338-43. Available from: https://pubmed.ncbi.nlm.nih.gov/23453102/

[11] Bernat I, Horak D, Stasek J. et al. 2014. "ST-segment elevation myocardial infarction treated by radial or femoral approach in a multicenter randomized clinical trial: The STEMI-RADIAL trial." *J Am Coll Cardio* 63 (10): 964-72

[12] Le May, M, Wells, G, So D et al. 2020. "Safety and Efficacy of Femoral Access vs Radial Access in ST-Segment Elevation Myocardial Infarction: The SAFARI-STEMI Randomized Clinical." *JAMA Cardiol* 5 (2): 126-34.

[13] Shiloh AL, Savel RH, Paulin LM, Eisen LA. 2011. "Ultrasound-guided catheterization of the radial artery: a systematic review and meta-analysis of randomized controlled trials." *CHEST* 139 (3): 524-29

[14] Kumar CS, Chugh S, Chugh Y et al. 2013. ". Feasibility and utility of pre-procedure ultrasound imaging of the arm to facilitate transradial coronary diagnostic and interventional procedures (PRIMAFACIE-TRI)." *Catheter Cardiiovasc Interv* 82 (1): 64-73.

[15] Seto AH, Roberts JS, Abu-Fadel MS et al. 2015. "Real-time ultrasound guidance facilitates transradial access: RAUST (Radial Artery Access with Ultrasound Trial)." *JACC Cardiovasc Interv* 8 (2): 283-91.

[16] Nguyen P, Makris A, Hennessy A et al. 2019. "Standard versus ultrasound-guided radial and femoral access in coronary angiography and intervention (SURF): a randomised controlled trial." *EuroIntervention* 15 (6): e522-30.

[17] Abazid RM, Sm=ettie OA, Mohamed MZ et al. 2017. "Radial artery ultrasound predicts the success of transradial coronary angiography." *Cardiol J* 24 (1): 9-14.

[18] Bernat I, Aminian A, Pancholy S et al. 2019. "Best Practices for the Prevention of Radial Artery Occlusion After Transradial Diagnostic Angiography and Intervention: An International Consensus Paper." *JACC: Cardio Interv* 12: 235-46.

[19] Rashid M, Kwok CS, Pancholy S, Chugh S, Kedev SA, Bernat I, et al. Radial artery occlusion after transradial interventions: A systematic review and meta-analysis. J Am Heart Assoc [Internet]. 2016 Jan 1 [cited 2020 Sep 27];5(1). Available from: https://www.ahajournals.org/doi/10.1161/JAHA.115.002686

[20] Hahalis GN, Leopoulou M, Tsigkas G et al. 2018. "Multicenter Randomized Evaluation of High Versus Standard Heparin Dose on Incident Radial Arterial Occlusion After Transradial Coronary Angiography: The SPIRIT OF ARTEMIS Study." *JACC Cardiovasc Interv* 26 (11): 2241-50.

[21] Shroff AR, Gulatis R, Drachmann DE et al. 2020. "SCAI expert consensus staement update on best practices for transradial angiography and itnervention." *Catheter Cardiovasc Interv* 95 (2): 245-52.

[22] Horie K, Tada N, Isawa T et al. 2018. "A randomised comparison of incidence of radial artery occlusion and symptomatic radial artery spasm associated with elective transradial coronary intervention using 6.5 Fr SheathLess Eaucath Guiding Catheter vs. 6.0 Fr Glidesheath Slender." *EuroIntervent* 17: 2018-25

[23] Amianian A, Saito S, Takahashi A et al. 2017. "Comparison of a new slender 6F sheath with a standard 5F sheath for transradial coronary angiography and intervention: RAP and BEAT (Radial Artery Patency and Bleeding, Efficacy, Adverse eventT), a randomized multicentre trial." *Eurointervention* 13 (5): e549-56.

[24] Chen Y, Ke Z, Xiao J et al. Subcutaneous Injection of Nitroglycerin at the Radial Artery Puncture Site Reduces the Risk of Early Radial Artery Occlusion After Transradial Coronary Catheterization 2018. *Circ Cardiovasc Interv* 11 (7): e006571.

[25] Pancholy S, Coppola J, Patel T et al. 2008. "Prevention of radial artery occlusion - Patent Hemostasis Evaluation Trial (PROPHET study): A randomized comparison of traditional versus patency documented hemostasis after transradial catheterization." *Catheter Cardiovasc Interv* 72 (3): 335-40.

[26] Pancholy S, Bernat I, Bertrand OF. 2016. "Prevention of Radial Artery Occlusion After Transradial Catheterization: The PROPHET-II Randomized Trial." *JACC: Cardiovasc Interven* 9 (19): 1992-99.

[27] Abdelaal E, Brousseau-Provencher C, Montiminy S, et al. 2013. "Risk Score, Causes and Clinical Impact of Falure of Transrdial Approach for Percutaneous Coroanry Interventions." *JACC: Cardiovasc Interv* 6 (11): 1129-37.

[28] Kwan TW, Ratcliffe JA, Huang Y et al. 2012. "Balloon-assisted sheathless

transradial intervention (BASTI) using 5Fr guiding catheters." *J Invasive Cardiol* 24 (5): 231-33.

[29] Coscas R, de Blic, R, Capdevila C et al. 2015. "Percutaneous radial access for peripheral transluminal angioplasty." *J Vasc Surg* 61 (2): 463-68.

[30] Kumar AJ, Johnes LE, Kollmeyer KR et al. 2017. "Radial artery access for peripheral endovascular procedures." J Vasc Surg 66 (3): 820-25.

[31] Hung ML, Lee EW, McWilliams JP et al. 2019. "A reality check in transradial access: a single-centre comparison of transradial and trasnfermoral access for abdominal and peripheral intervention." *European Radiology* 29: 68-74.

[32] Posham R, Young LB, Lookstein RA et al. 2018. "Radial Access for Lower Extremity Peripheral Arterial Interventions: Do we Have teh Tools?" *Semin Intervent Radiol* 35 (5): 427-34.

[33] Terashima M, Meguro Taiichiro, Takeda H et al. 2001. "Percutaneous ulnar artery approach for coronary angiography: A preliminary report in nine patients." *Cathet Cardiovasc Interven* 53 (3): 410-14.

[34] Dashkoff N, Dashkoff PT, Zizzi JA et al. 2002. "Ulnar artery cannulation for coronary nagiography and percutaensou coronary intervention: Case reports adn anatomic considerations." *Catheter Cardiovasc Interv* 55 (1): 93-96.

[35] Layton KF, Kallmes DF and Kaufmann TJ. 2006. "Use of the Ulnar Artery asa an Alternative Access Site for Cerebra Angiography." *ANJR* 27 (10): 2073-74.

[36] Daal K, Rijal J, Lee J et al. 2016. "Transulnar versus transradial access for cornaronay angoigraphy or percutanesou coroanry intervetion: A meta-analysis of randomzied controlled trials." *Catheter Cardioavasc Interv* 87 (5): 857-65.

[37] Hahalis G, Tsigkas G, Xanthopoulou I et al. 2013. "Transulnar Compared with Transradial Artery Approach as a Default Stragegy for Coronary Procedure." *Circulation: Cardiovasc Interv* 6 (3): 252-61.

[38] Gaudino M, Benedetto U, Fremes S et al. 2020. "Association of Radial Artery Graft vs Saphenous Vein Graft wiht Long -Term Cardiovascular Outcomes among Patients Undersgoing Coronary Artery Bypass Grafting: A systematic REview and Meta-Analysis." *JAMA* 324 (2): 179-87.

[39] Kamiya H, Ushijima T, Kanamori T et al. 2003. "Use of the radial artery graft after transradial catheterization: is it suitable as a bypass conduit?" *Ann Thoac Surg* 76 (5): 1505-09.

[40] Burstein JM, Gidrewicz D, Hutchison SJ et al. 2007. "Impact of radial artery cannulation for coronary angiography and agnioplasty on radial artery function." *Am J Cardiol* 99 (4): 457-59.

[41] Dawson EA, Rathore S, Cable NT et al. 2010. "Impact of Introducer Sheath Coating on endothelial Function in Humans After Transradial Coroanry Procedures." *Circ Cardiovasc Interv* 3: 148-56.

[42] Di Vito L, Burzotta F, Trani C et al. 2014. "Radial artery complications occuring after transradial coroanry procedures using long hydrophylic-coated introducer sheath: a frequency domain-opitcal cohenence tomography study." *Int J Cardiovasc Imaging* 30: 21-29.

[43] Klein LW, Goldstein JA, Haines D et al. 2020. "SCAI Multi-Society Position Statement on Occupational Health Hazards of hte Catheterization Laboratory: Shifting the Paradigm for Healthcare Workers' Protection." *JACC* 75 (14): 1718-24.

[44] Tesfaldet MT, Mohammed A, Aristoltelis P et al. 2013. "A Randomized

Comparison of the Transradial and Transfemoral Approaches for Coronary Artery Bypass Graft Angiography and Intervention: The RADIAL-CABG Trial (RADIAL Versus Femoral Access for Coronary Artery Bypass Graft Angiography and Intervention)." *JACC* 6 (11): 1138-44.

[45] Sciahbasi A, Romagnoli E, Burzotta R et al. 2011. "Transradial approach (left vs right) and procedural times during percutaneous coronary procedures: TALENT study." *Am Heart J* 161 (1): 172-79.

[46] Shah B, Burdowski J, Guo Y et al. 2016. "Effect of Left Versus Right Radial Artery Approach for Coronary Angiography on Radiation Parameters in Patients With Predictors of Transradial Access Failure." *Am J Cardi* 118 (4): 447-81.

[47] Dominici M, Diletti R, Milici C et al. 2013. "Operator exposure to x-ray in left and right radial access during percutaneous coronary procedures: OPERA randomised study." *Heart* 99: 480-84.

[48] Norgas T, Gorgulu S and Dagdelen S. 2012. "A randomized study comparing the effectiveness of right and left radial approach for coronary angiography." *Catheter Cardiovasc Interv* 80 (2): 260-64.

[49] Kado H, Patel AM, Suryadevera S et al "Operator Radiation Exposure and Physical Discomfort During a Right Versus Left Radial Approach for Coronary Interventions A Randomized Evaluation" JACC: Cardiovasc Interv 2014: 810-14

[50] Pancholy S, Joshi P, Shah S et al. 2015. "Effect of Vascular Access Site Choice on Radiation Exposure During Coronary Angiography." *JACC: Cardvasc Interv* 8 (9): 1189-96.

[51] Fiorilli PN, Kobayashi T, Giri J, Hirshfield JW. 2019. "Strategies for radiation exposure-sparing in fluoroscopically guided invasive cardiovascular procedures." *Catheter Cardiovasc Interv* 95 (1): 118-127.

[52] Panetta CJ, Galbraith EM, Yanavitski M et al. 2020. "Reduced radiation exposure in the cardiac catheterization laboratory with a novel vertical radiation shield." *Catheter Cardiovasc Interv* 95 (1): 7-12.

[53] Mehta SK, Frutkin AD, Lindsey JB et al. 2009. "Bleeding in patients undergoing percutaneous coronary intervention: the development of a clinical risk algorithm from the National Cardiovascular Data Registry." *Circ Cardiovasc Interv* 2 (3): 222-29.

[54] Piper WD, Malenka DJ, Ryan TJ et al. 2003. "Predicting vascular complications in percutaneous coronary interventions." *Am Heart J* 145 (6): 1022-29.

[55] Secco GG, Marinucci L, Uguccioni L et al. 2013. "Transradial versus transfemoral approach for primary percutaneous coronary interventions in elderly patients." 25 (5): 254-46.

[56] Cantor WJ, Mehta SR, MMath FY et al. 2015. "Radial versus femoral access for elderly patients with acute coronary syndrome undergoing coronary angiography and intervention: insights from the RIVAL trial." *Am Heart J* 170 (5): 880-86.

Section 2

Percutaneous Valve Replacement

Chapter 4

The Current Perspectives in Valve-in-Valve Transcatheter Aortic Valve Replacement

Takashi Murashita

Abstract

The increased use of bioprostheses in aortic valve replacement has led to increased number of patients with structural valve degeneration. Since reoperation for failed bioprostheses carries a high risk, a valve-in-valve transcatheter aortic valve replacement has become an attractive alternative treatment. However, there remains technical challenges and controversies in this field. Herein, we discuss the current perspectives in valve-in-valve transcatheter aortic valve replacement.

Keywords: transcatheter aortic valve replacement, valve-in-valve, failed bioprostheses

1. Introduction

The use of bioprosthetic valves in aortic valve replacement (AVR) has been increasing, even in younger patients [1]. In the meantime, the indication of transcatheter aortic valve replacement (TAVR) has been expanding as well. Since reoperation for degenerated prosthetic valve carries a high risk, a valve-in-valve TAVR has become an attractive alternative treatment. The most recent guidelines stated that valve-in-valve TAVR is recommended as class IIa indication for "severely symptomatic patients with bioprosthetic aortic valve stenosis judged by the heart team to be at high or prohibitive risk of reoperation, and in whom improvement in hemodynamics is anticipated" [2]. However, technical challenges exist in valve-in-valve TAVR. In this chapter, we discuss the current perspective of valve-in-valve TAVR and its associated risks and benefits.

2. Indications of valve-in-valve TAVR

2.1 Outcomes of redo aortic valve replacement

The use of bioprosthetic valve in AVR has been expanding. That will inevitably lead to increased number of patients who need re-aortic valve replacement for degenerated bioprostheses. Redo aortic valve replacement carries a higher operative risk compared to primary aortic valve replacement.

Kaneko et al. investigated 3,380 patients from The Society of Thoracic Surgeons database who underwent elective, isolated redo aortic valve replacement (AVR) after a previous AVR [3]. The operative mortality was 4.6%, and the incidence of

Study	Year	Number of pts	Key outcomes
Dvir et al. [4]	2014	459	Thirty-day mortality; 7.6%. Thirty-day stroke rate; 1.7%. One-year survival rate; 83.2%. Patients who had stenosis had worse 1-year survival in comparison with regurgitation. Patients with small valves had worse 1-year survival in comparison with intermediate or large valves.
Tuzcu et al. [5]	2018	1150	Thirty-day mortality; 2.9%. Thirty-day stroke rate; 1.7%. Thirty-day heart failure hospitalization rate; 2.4%. One-year survival rate; 88.3%. Patients in the valve-in-valve TAVR group had higher post-TAVR mean gradient, but less moderate or severe aortic regurgitation compared to native-valve TAVR group. Post-TAVR gradients were highest in small SAVRs and stenotic SAVRs.
Webb et al. [6]	2017	365	Thirty-day mortality; 2.7%. Thirty-day stroke rate; 2.7%. One-year survival rate; 87.6%. Mean transaortic gradient was 17.6 mm Hg, and effective orifice area was 1.16 cm^2 at 1 year.
Webb et al. [7]	2019	365	Three-year survival rate; 67.3% Aortic valve re-replacement was required in 1.9%. Mean transaortic gradient was 16.6 mm Hg at 3-year follow-up. Effective orifice area was 1.15 cm^2 at 3-year follow-up. Moderate to severe aortic regurgitation was 2.5% at 3 years. New York Heart Association functional class improved, with 90.4% in class III or IV at baseline and 14.1% at 3 years.
Neupane et al. [8]	2018	227	Thirty-day mortality; 5%. Thirty-day major stroke rate; 2%. Permanent pacemaker implantation; 9%. Valve-in-valve TAVR and re-SAVR had similar thirty-day mortality, and similar rates of stroke, myocardial infarction, and acute kidney injury requiring dialysis.
Pibarot et al. [9]	2018	1168	Thirty-day mortality; 10.3% in severe PPM, 4.3% in no or moderate PPM. Adjusted one-year survival rate; 80.7% in severe PPM, 89.1% in no or moderate PPM. Patients with pre-existing severe PPM more frequently harbored high post-procedural gradients.

Study	Year	Number of pts	Key outcomes
Deeb et al. [10]	2017	227	Thirty-day mortality; 2.2%. Thirty-day major stroke rate; 0.4%. One-year survival rate; 85.4%. Moderate aortic regurgitation occurred in 3.5% of patients at 30 days and 7.4% of patients at 1 year, with no severe aortic regurgitation. The rate of new permanent pacemaker implantation was 8.1% at 30 days and 11.0% at 1 year. The mean valve gradient was 17.0 ± 8.8 mm Hg at 30 days and 16.6 ± 8.9 mm Hg at 1 year. Factors significantly associated with higher discharge mean aortic gradients were surgical valve size, stenosis as modality of surgical valve failure, and presence of surgical valve prosthesis patient mismatch.
de Freitas Campos Guimarães et ak [11]	2018	116	Thirty-day mortality; 6.9%. Three-year survival rate; 74.1%. Average mean transaortic gradients remained stable up to 5-year follow-up. Clinically relevant structural valve degeneration occurred in 3%, and 15.1% had subclinical structural valve degeneration.
Goztek et al. [12]	2018	342	Thirty-day mortality; 5.4%. Permanent pacemaker implantation; 6.8%. Valve-in-valve TAVR was associated with higher incidence of PPM, higher paravalvular leaks and higher mean postoperative aortic valve gradients compared to re-SAVR.

TAVR: transcatheter aortic valve replacement; SAVR: surgical aortic valve replacement; PPM: prosthesis-patient mismatch.

Table 1.
Previous studies which reported the clinical outcomes of valve-in-valve TAVR.

mortality, morbidity, stroke, postoperative aortic insufficiency mild or greater, pacemaker implantation and vascular complications was higher in redo AVR group compared to primary AVR patients.

2.2 Outcomes of valve-in-valve TAVR

Overall the outcomes of valve-in-valve TAVR have been reported to equivalent or better compared to those of redo surgical AVR.

The Valve-in-Valve International Data (VIVID) reported the outcomes of valve-in-valve TAVR for 459 patients in 55 centers [4]. The thirty-day mortality was 7.6%. Overall one-year survival rate was 83.2% Patients with bioprosthetic stenosis had worse 1-year survival compared with the patients with bioprosthetic regurgitation. Patients with small valves had worse 1-year survival compared to intermediate or large valves.

The Transcatheter Valve Therapy (TVT) Registry showed that unadjusted 30-day mortality after valve-in-valve TAVR was 2.9%, and it was better than that of native valve TAVR (4.8%) [5].

The PARTNER (Placement of Aortic Transcatheter Valves) 2 trial showed that 30-day mortality was 2.7%, stroke was 2.7%, major vascular complication was 4.1%, conversion to surgery was 0.6%, coronary occlusion was 0.8%, new pacemaker insertion was 1.9%, and one year all-cause mortality was 12.4% [6]. Recently 3-year outcomes after valve-in-valve TAVR in the Partner 2 registry was published [7]. The mean age of the patients was 78.9 ± 10.2 years. At 3 years, the estimate all-cause mortality was 32.7%. Quality of life of the patients improved compared to baseline.

Neupane et al. conducted a meta-analysis of the previously reported studies to determine outcomes after valve-in-valve TAVR and redo AVR [8]. Their analysis showed no difference in 30-day mortality between valve-in-valve TAVR and redo AVR for failed bioprosthetic aortic valve.

Previous studies which reported the clinical outcomes of valve-in-valve TAVR are listed in **Table 1**.

3. Complications in valve-in-valve TAVR

3.1 Prosthesis-patient mismatch

Valve-in-valve TAVR could cause prosthesis-patient mismatch especially when there was severe bioprosthetic valve stenosis. It was also pointed out that valve-in-valve TAVR was an independent predictor of valve hemodynamic deterioration (defined as an increase in mean aortic valve gradient ≥10 mm Hg) [13].

Herrmann et al. reviewed 62,125 patients in the Society of Thoracic Surgeons/American College of Cardiology TVT registry and reported that severe prosthesis-patient mismatch occurred in 12% [14]. Patients with severe prosthesis-patient mismatch had higher mortality rate compared to patients with moderate or no prosthesis-patient mismatch.

On the contrary, Dvir et al. reported that severe prosthesis-patient mismatch occurred in 31.8% of patients surviving aortic valve-in-valve TAVR [4]. However, one-year survival was not affected by having severe prosthesis-patient mismatch.

The long-term transaortic gradient has not been reported. In the Partner II registry, mean transaortic gradient was 16.6 mmHg at 3-year follow-up [7].

3.2 Coronary obstruction

Coronary obstruction is a rare, but life-threatening complication associated with TAVR. Its incidence in native valve TAVR was reported as less than 1% [15]. However, it occurs more frequently in valve-in-valve TAVR.

Ribeiro et al. reviewed 1,612 patients from the Valve-in-Valve International Data Registry [16]. Coronary obstruction occurred in 37 patients (2.3%), and the 30-day mortality was 52.9% among the patients who had coronary obstruction. Coronary obstruction happened more frequently in stented valves with externally mounted leaflets or stentless valves compared to stented valves with internally mounted leaflets.

Multiple detector computed tomography is a standard diagnostic modality in the planning of TAVR [17]. A virtual transcatheter valve to coronary ostium distance <4 mm is considered a high risk of coronary obstruction [16].

In the case of anticipated high risk of coronary obstruction, a placement of a coronary guidewire with coronary balloon or undeployed stent in the targeted coronary arteries before deploying TAVR is a good option for coronary protection, since the emergent percutaneous coronary intervention for coronary obstruction is challenging. Ribeiro et al. reported that percutaneous coronary intervention was successful only in 81.8% [15].

Delayed coronary obstruction is a rare complication following TAVR that accompanies with high in-hospital mortality. Jabbour et al. reported that the incidence of delayed coronary obstruction was 0.22% in 17,092 TAVR procedures and the overall in-hospital mortality was 50% [18]. Percutaneous coronary intervention was successful only in 68.8%. It occurred more frequently after valve-in-valve TAVR compared to native valve TAVR (0.89% vs. 0.18%) and it occurred more frequently in self-expandable valves compared to balloon-expandable valves (0.36% vs. 0.11%).

3.3 Self-expandable valve versus balloon-expandable valve

Self-expanding valves are usually associated with lower postprocedural gradients. Rogers et al. reported that hemodynamics of self-expandable valves were superior to that of balloon-expandable valves in patients with small aortic annulus [19].

In the meantime, Dvir et al. reported that elevated postprocedural gradients were happened more frequently in balloon expandable valves compared with self-expandable valves [4].

Pibarot et al. reported that pre-existing prosthesis-patient mismatch of the failed surgical valve was strongly and independently associated with increased risk for mortality following valve-in-valve TAVR [9]. Elevated pressure gradients are seen in more than 70% of patients who present with baseline prosthesis-patient mismatch if treated with balloon-expandable valves.

The optimal deployment height would be important to avoid postprocedural high gradients. Simonato et al. reported that lower gradients and greater effective orifice areas were achieved with higher deployment positions than lower deployment in vitro study [20]. Hatoum et al. reported that supra-annular axial deployment is associated with lower pressure gradients, and sub-annular deployment is associated with more favorable sinus hemodynamics [21].

When severe prosthesis-patient mismatch is present, a self-expanding device in a supra-annular position would be the preferred treatment strategy. Dvir et al. suggested an implant depth of up to 3 mm for the self-expandable valve; Evolut (Medtronic, Minneapolis, Minnesota), and up to 20% frame depth for the balloon-expandable valve; SAPIEN 3 (Edwards Lifesciences, Irvine, California) [22].

3.4 Structural valve deterioration after TAVR

Bioprosthetic valve dysfunction happens both in surgical AVR and TAVR. However, bioprosthetic valve dysfunction is a broad term that encompasses structural and non-structural valve deterioration [23]. It is very important to distinguish between two of them. Structural valve deterioration is the principal etiological factor, and it can lead to irreversible valve dysfunction, whereas non-structural valve deterioration includes reversible dysfunction such as valve thrombosis or endocarditis.

The long-term durability of valve-in-valve TAVR has been unknown. One of the longest follow-up data was reported from Partner II registry [7]. Among 337 patients who could be followed for 3 years, 5 patients underwent repeat aortic valve replacement for aortic valve dysfunction after valve-in-valve procedure. Moderate hemodynamic valve deterioration occurred in 2 out of 160 patients

(1.3%), and severe hemodynamic valve deterioration also occurred in 2 out of 160patients (1.3%) at 3 years.

3.5 Valve thrombosis

Valve thrombosis following TAVR has been increasingly recognized. Valve thrombosis is associated with reduced leaflet motion, and leads to high chance of strokes and transient ischemic attacks. Subclinical leaflet thrombosis is manifested by either hypo-attenuated leaflet thickening or reduced leaflet motion [24].

Del Trigo et al. reported that the incidence of valve hemodynamic deterioration following TAVR was 4.5% in 1,521 patients, and a valve-in-valve procedure was an independent predictor for valve hemodynamic deterioration [25].

Vahidkhah et al. analyzed computational three-dimensional models for the surgical aortic valve and transcatheter aortic valve [26]. They found that geometric confinement of the transcather aortic valve by the leaflets and the frame of the degenerated bioprosthesis that circumferentially surround the transcatheter aortic valve stent increased the blood residence time on the leaflets, which could act as a permissive factor in the leaflet thrombosis after valve-in-valve TAVR.

3.6 Antiplatelet/anticoagulation therapy after TAVR

The optimal antiplatelet/anticoagulation management after TAVR has been controversial [23, 27].

Most of the societies such as American Heart Association and Society of Thoracic Surgeons recommend lifelong-aspirin and 6 months of Clopidogrel after TAVR. In terms of anticoagulant therapy, it may be considered in patients with chronic atrial fibrillation or other indications. Vitamin K antagonist may be considered in the first 3 months after procedure in patients at risk for atrial fibrillation or valve thrombosis.

Overtchouk et al. reviewed 11,469 patients in French registry, and found that anticoagulation decreased the risk of bioprosthetic valve dysfunction, whereas chronic renal failure and prosthesis size ≤23 mm were associated with the risk of bioprosthetic valve dysfunction [28].

4. Conclusions

The valve-in-valve TAVR has provided satisfactory outcomes for degenerative bioprosthetic aortic valve. It is recommended with class IIa indication in high risk patients for redo surgical AVR. However, physicians need to understand technical challenges in valve-in-valve TAVR such as residual high pressure gradient, prosthesis-patient mismatch and coronary obstruction. The long-term durability of valve-in-valve procedure remains unknown. Moreover, anticoagulation management and superiority between self-expandable and balloon-expandable valves have been controversial.

Author details

Takashi Murashita
University of Missouri, Columbia, Missouri, USA

Address all correspondence to: tmurashita@gmail.com

References

[1] Brown JM, O'Brien SM, Wu C, Sikora JA, Griffith BP, Gammie JS. Isolated aortic valve replacement in North America comprising 108,687 patients in 10 years: changes in risks, valve types, and outcomes in the Society of Thoracic Surgeons National Database. J Thorac Cardiovasc Surg. 2009;137:82-90. DOI: 10.1016/j.jtcvs.2008.08.015

[2] Nishimura RA, Otto CM, Bonow RO, Carabello BA, Erwin JP 3rd, Fleisher LA, Jneid H, Mack MJ, McLeod CJ, O'Gara PT, Rigolin VH, Sundt TM 3rd, Thompson A. 2017 AHA/ACC Focused Update of the 2014 AHA/ACC Guideline for the Management of Patients With Valvular Heart Disease: A Report of the American College of Cardiology/American Heart Association Task Force on Clinical Practice Guidelines. Circulation. 2017;135:1159-1195. DOI: 10.1161/CIR.0000000000000503

[3] Kaneko T, Vassileva CM, Englum B, Kim S, Yammine M, Brennan M, Suri RM, Thourani VH, Jacobs JP, Aranki S. Contemporary Outcomes of Repeat Aortic Valve Replacement: A Benchmark for Transcatheter Valve-in-Valve Procedures. Ann Thorac Surg. 2015;100:1298-1304. DOI: 10.1016/j.athoracsur.2015.04.062

[4] Dvir D, Webb JG, Bleiziffer S, Pasic M, Waksman R, Kodali S, Barbanti M, Latib A, Schaefer U, Rodés-Cabau J, Treede H, Piazza N, Hildick-Smith D, Himbert D, Walther T, Hengstenberg C, Nissen H, Bekeredjian R, Presbitero P, Ferrari E, Segev A, de Weger A, Windecker S, Moat NE, Napodano M, Wilbring M, Cerillo AG, Brecker S, Tchetche D, Lefèvre T, De Marco F, Fiorina C, Petronio AS, Teles RC, Testa L, Laborde JC, Leon MB, Kornowski R; Valve-in-Valve International Data Registry Investigators. Transcatheter aortic valve implantation in failed bioprosthetic surgical valves. JAMA. 2014;312:162-170. DOI: 10.1001/jama.2014.7246

[5] Tuzcu EM, Kapadia SR, Vemulapalli S, Carroll JD, Holmes DR Jr, Mack MJ, Thourani VH, Grover FL, Brennan JM, Suri RM, Dai D, Svensson LG. Transcatheter Aortic Valve Replacement of Failed Surgically Implanted Bioprostheses: The STS/ACC Registry. J Am Coll Cardiol. 2018;72:370-382. DOI: 10.1016/j.jacc.2018.04.074

[6] Webb JG, Mack MJ, White JM, Dvir D, Blanke P, Herrmann HC, Leipsic J, Kodali SK, Makkar R, Miller DC, Pibarot P, Pichard A, Satler LF, Svensson L, Alu MC, Suri RM, Leon MB. Transcatheter Aortic Valve Implantation Within Degenerated Aortic Surgical Bioprostheses: PARTNER 2 Valve-in-Valve Registry. J Am Coll Cardiol. 2017;69:2253-2262. DOI: 10.1016/j.jacc.2017.02.057

[7] Webb JG, Murdoch DJ, Alu MC, Cheung A, Crowley A, Dvir D, Herrmann HC, Kodali SK, Leipsic J, Miller DC, Pibarot P, Suri RM, Wood D, Leon MB, Mack MJ. 3-Year Outcomes After Valve-in-Valve Transcatheter Aortic Valve Replacement for Degenerated Bioprostheses: The PARTNER 2 Registry. J Am Coll Cardiol. 2019;73:2647-2655. DOI: 10.1016/j.jacc.2019.03.483

[8] Neupane S, Singh H, Lämmer J, Othman H, Yamasaki H, Rosman HS, Bossone E, Mehta RH, Eggebrecht H. Meta-Analysis of Transcatheter Valve-in-Valve Implantation Versus Redo Aortic Valve Surgery for Bioprosthetic Aortic Valve Dysfunction. Am J Cardiol 2018;212:1593-1600. DOI: 10.1016/j.amjcard.2018.02.054

[9] Pibarot P, Simonato M, Barbanti M, Linke A, Kornowski R, Rudolph T,

Spence M, Moat N, Aldea G, Mennuni M, Iadanza A, Amrane H, Gaia D, Kim WK, Napodano M, Baumbach H, Finkelstein A, Kobayashi J, Brecker S, Don C, Cerillo A, Unbehaun A, Attias D, Nejjari M, Jones N, Fiorina C, Tchetche D, Philippart R, Spargias K, Hernandez JM, Latib A, Dvir D. Impact of Pre-Existing Prosthesis-Patient Mismatch on Survival Following Aortic Valve-in-Valve Procedures. JACC Cardiovasc Interv. 2018;11:133-141. DOI: 10.1016/j.jcin.2017.08.039

[10] Deeb GM, Chetcuti SJ, Reardon MJ, Patel HJ, Grossman PM, Schreiber T, Forrest JK, Bajwa TK, O'Hair DP, Petrossian G, Robinson N, Katz S, Hartman A, Dauerman HL, Schmoker J, Khabbaz K, Watson DR, Yakubov SJ, Oh JK, Li S, Kleiman NS, Adams DH, Popma JJ. 1-Year Results in Patients Undergoing Transcatheter Aortic Valve Replacement With Failed Surgical Bioprostheses. JACC Cardiovasc Interv. 2017;10:1034-1044. DOI: 10.1016/j.jcin.2017.03.018

[11] de Freitas Campos Guimarães L, Urena M, Wijeysundera HC, Munoz-Garcia A, Serra V, Benitez LM, Auffret V, Cheema AN, Amat-Santos IJ, Fisher Q, Himbert D, Garcia Del Blanco B, Dager A, Le Breton H, Paradis JM, Dumont E, Pibarot P, Rodés-Cabau J. Long-Term Outcomes After Transcatheter Aortic Valve-in-Valve Replacement. Circ Cardiovasc Interv. 2018;11:e007038. DOI: 10.1161/CIRCINTERVENTIONS.118.007038

[12] Gozdek M, Raffa GM, Suwalski P, Kolodziejczak M, Anisimowicz L, Kubica J, Navarese EP, Kowalewski M; SIRIO-TAVI group. Comparative performance of transcatheter aortic valve-in-valve implantation versus conventional surgical redo aortic valve replacement in patients with degenerated aortic valve bioprostheses: systematic review and meta-analysis. Eur J Cardiothorac Surg. 2018;53:495-504. DOI: 10.1093/ejcts/ezx347.

[13] Vemulapalli S, Holmes DR Jr, Dai D, Matsouaka R, Mack MJ, Grover FL, Makkar RR, Thourani VH, Douglas PS. Valve hemodynamic deterioration and cardiovascular outcomes in TAVR: A report from the STS/ACC TVT Registry. Am Heart J. 2018;195:1-13. DOI: 10.1016/j.ahj.2017.09.005

[14] Herrmann HC, Daneshvar SA, Fonarow GC, Stebbins A, Vemulapalli S, Desai ND, Malenka DJ, Thourani VH, Rymer J, Kosinski AS. Prosthesis-Patient Mismatch in Patients Undergoing Transcatheter Aortic Valve Replacement: From the STS/ACC TVT Registry. J Am Coll Cardiol. 2018;72:2701-2711. DOI: 10.1016/j.jacc.2018.09.001

[15] Ribeiro HB, Webb JG, Makkar RR, Cohen MG, Kapadia SR, Kodali S, Tamburino C, Barbanti M, Chakravarty T, Jilaihawi H, Paradis JM, de Brito FS Jr, Cánovas SJ, Cheema AN, de Jaegere PP, del Valle R, Chiam PT, Moreno R, Pradas G, Ruel M, Salgado-Fernández J, Sarmento-Leite R, Toeg HD, Velianou JL, Zajarias A, Babaliaros V, Cura F, Dager AE, Manoharan G, Lerakis S, Pichard AD, Radhakrishnan S, Perin MA, Dumont E, Larose E, Pasian SG, Nombela-Franco L, Urena M, Tuzcu EM, Leon MB, Amat-Santos IJ, Leipsic J, Rodés-Cabau J. Predictive factors, management, and clinical outcomes of coronary obstruction following transcatheter aortic valve implantation: insights from a large multicenter registry. J Am Coll Cardiol 2013;62:1552-1562. DOI: 10.1016/j.jacc.2013.07.040

[16] Ribeiro HB, Rodés-Cabau J, Blanke P, Leipsic J, Kwan Park J, Bapat V, Makkar R, Simonato M, Barbanti M, Schofer J, Bleiziffer S, Latib A, Hildick-Smith D, Presbitero P, Windecker S, Napodano M, Cerillo AG, Abdel-Wahab M, Tchetche D, Fiorina C,

Sinning JM, Cohen MG, Guerrero ME, Whisenant B, Nietlispach F, Palma JH, Nombela-Franco L, de Weger A, Kass M, Sandoli de Brito F Jr, Lemos PA, Kornowski R, Webb J, Dvir D. Incidence, predictors, and clinical outcomes of coronary obstruction following transcatheter aortic valve replacement for degenerative bioprosthetic surgical valves: insights from the VIVID registry. Eur Heart J 2018;39:687-695. DOI: 10.1093/eurheartj/ehx455

[17] Blanke P, Weir-McCall JR, Achenbach S, Delgado V, Hausleiter J, Jilaihawi H, Marwan M, Nørgaard BL, Piazza N, Schoenhagen P, Leipsic JA. Computed Tomography Imaging in the Context of Transcatheter Aortic Valve Implantation (TAVI)/Transcatheter Aortic Valve Replacement (TAVR): An Expert Consensus Document of the Society of Cardiovascular Computed Tomography. JACC Cardiovasc Imaging. 2019;12:1-24. DOI: 10.1016/j.jcmg.2018.12.003

[18] Jabbour RJ, Tanaka A, Finkelstein A, Mack M, Tamburino C, Van Mieghem N, de Backer O, Testa L, Gatto P, Purita P, Rahhab Z, Veulemans V, Stundl A, Barbanti M, Nerla R, Sinning JM, Dvir D, Tarantini G, Szerlip M, Scholtz W, Scholtz S, Tchetche D, Castriota F, Butter C, Søndergaard L, Abdel-Wahab M, Sievert H, Alfieri O, Webb J, Rodés-Cabau J, Colombo A, Latib A. Delayed Coronary Obstruction After Transcatheter Aortic Valve Replacement. J Am Coll Cardiol. 2018;71:1513-1524. DOI: 10.1016/j.jacc.2018.01.066

[19] Rogers T, Steinvil A, Gai J, Torguson R, Koifman E, Kiramijyan S, Negi S, Lee SY, Okubagzi P, Satler LF, Ben-Dor I, Pichard AD, Waksman R. Choice of Balloon-Expandable Versus Self-Expanding Transcatheter Aortic Valve Impacts Hemodynamics Differently According to Aortic Annular Size. Am J Cardiol. 2017;119:900-904. DOI: 10.1016/j.amjcard.2016.11.044

[20] Simonato M, Azadani AN, Webb J, Leipsic J, Kornowski R, Vahanian A, Wood D, Piazza N, Kodali S, Ye J, Whisenant B, Gaia D, Aziz M, Pasala T, Mehilli J, Wijeysundera HC, Tchetche D, Moat N, Teles R, Petronio AS, Hildick-Smith D, Landes U, Windecker S, Arbel Y, Mendiz O, Makkar R, Tseng E, Dvir D. In vitro evaluation of implantation depth in valve-in-valve using different transcatheter heart valves. EuroIntervention 2016;12:909-917. DOI: 10.4244/EIJV12I7A149

[21] Hatoum H, Dollery J, Lilly SM, Crestanello JA, Dasi LP. Implantation Depth and Rotational Orientation Effect on Valve-in-Valve Hemodynamics and Sinus Flow. Ann Thorac Surg. 2018;106:70-78. DOI: 10.1016/j.athoracsur.2018.01.070

[22] Dvir D, Khan J, Kornowski R, Komatsu I, Chatriwalla A, Mackenson GB, Simonato M, Ribeiro H, Wood D, Leipsic J, Webb J, Mylotte D. Novel strategies in aortic valve-in-valve therapy including bioprosthetic valve fracture and BASILICA. EuroIntervention 2018;14:74-82. DOI: 10.4244/EIJ-D-18-00667

[23] Mazer CD, Bhatt DL, Verma S. Anticoagulation Following TAVR: No Clear Answer Yet. J Am Coll Cardiol. 2019;73:22-28. DOI: 10.1016/j.jacc.2018.11.012

[24] Yanagawa B, Mazine A, Bhatt DL, Clavel MA, Côté N, Cheema AN, Pibarot P, Verma S. Subclinical bioprosthetic aortic valve thrombosis: clinical and translational implications. Curr Opin Cardiol. 2017;32:137-146. DOI: 10.1097/HCO.0000000000000373

[25] Del Trigo M, Muñoz-Garcia AJ, Wijeysundera HC, Nombela-Franco L, Cheema AN, Gutierrez E, Serra V,

Kefer J, Amat-Santos IJ, Benitez LM, Mewa J, Jiménez-Quevedo P, Alnasser S, Garcia Del Blanco B, Dager A, Abdul-Jawad Altisent O, Puri R, Campelo-Parada F, Dahou A, Paradis JM, Dumont E, Pibarot P, Rodés-Cabau J. Incidence, Timing, and Predictors of Valve Hemodynamic Deterioration After Transcatheter Aortic Valve Replacement: Multicenter Registry. J Am Coll Cardiol. 2016;67:644-655. DOI: 10.1016/j.jacc.2015.10.097

[26] Vahidkhah K, Javani S, Abbasi M, Azadani PN, Tandar A, Dvir D, Azadani AN. Blood Stasis on Transcatheter Valve Leaflets and Implications for Valve-in-Valve Leaflet Thrombosis. Ann Thorac Surg. 2017;104:751-759. DOI: 10.1016/j.athoracsur.2017.02.052

[27] Sherwood MW. Vora AN. Challenges in Aortic Stenosis: Review of Antiplatelet/Anticoagulant Therapy Management with Transcatheter Aortic Valve Replacement (TAVR): TAVR with Recent PCI, TAVR in the Patient with Atrial Fibrillation, and TAVR Thrombosis Management. Curr Cardiol Rep. 2018;20:130. DOI: 10.1007/s11886-018-1073-9

[28] Overtchouk P, Guedeney P, Rouanet S, Verhoye JP, Lefevre T, Van Belle E, Eltchaninoff H, Gilard M, Leprince P, Iung B, Barthelemy O, Le Breton H, Souteyrand G, Vicaut E, Montalescot G, Collet JP. Long-Term Mortality and Early Valve Dysfunction According to Anticoagulation Use: The FRANCE TAVI Registry. J Am Coll Cardiol. 2019;73:13-21. DOI: 10.1016/j.jacc.2018.08.1045

Chapter 5

Transcatheter Mitral Valve Replacement: Evolution and Future Development

Lina Ya'qoub and Marvin Eng

Abstract

We will review transcatheter mitral valve replacement (TMVR) and discuss this evolving cutting edge procedure in terms of types (valve in valve, valve in ring and valve in mitral annular calcification MAC), clinical indications, pre-procedural planning and value of pre-procedural imaging including computed tomography role, technical challenges encountered in these procedures, potential complications for each type of TMVR, and potential strategies to mitigate and avoid such complications, We will review the currently available devices dedicated for mitral valve replacement, with a summary of their preliminary data and early outcome results. We will also discuss knowledge gaps and ideas for future research.

Keywords: Transcatheter mitral valve replacement, valve in valve, valve in ring, valve in mitral annular calcification

1. Introduction

Valvular heart disease affects >100 million patients worldwide, which is estimated to increase further with the aging population and a subsequent increase in degenerative valve disease [1]. Based on analysis of the Society of Thoracic Surgery (STS) National Database, there are >40,000 mitral valve replacements being performed annually in the United States (US), with shift from mechanical to bioprosthetic valve replacements [1]. It is known that redo mitral valve surgery is associated with higher mortality compared to first mitral surgery; with 30-day mortality ranging from 6% for elective second mitral valve surgery and 17.8% for emergency surgery [2]. The risk of a third or fourth surgery is even higher; with 30-day mortality reaching up to 44% in urgent surgery [3]. As such, Transcatheter mitral valve replacement (TMVR) using aortic balloon-expandable transcatheter heart valves (THV) has been increasingly performed for patients with severe mitral valve disease who are not candidates for surgery [4]; as it emerged as a less invasive alternative option for these patients with relatively lower mortality than the predicted STS predicted rates of mortality [4]. Moreover, dedicated devices for TMVR have been developed and some are currently being studied [5–10]. Results of the clinical outcomes of TMVR are promising, but anatomical differences between mitral bioprosthetic valves, annuloplasty rings, and severely calcified mitral annulus are associated with specific procedural challenges for TMVR procedures [1, 4].

2. Types of TMVR

There are three main types of TMVR: 1) valve-in-valve (ViV) for severe mitral valve disease due to degenerated mitral bioprosthetic valves, 2) valve-in-ring (ViR) for failed surgical repairs with annuloplasty rings, and 3) valve-in-mitral annular calcifications (ViMAC) for native mitral valve disease with severe MAC who are poor surgical candidates [1]. Mitral ViV for high surgical risk patients was approved by the Food and Drug Administration (FDA) in the United States (US) in 2017, while mitral ViR and ViMAC remain off-label at this current time [4]. The role of TMVR in native mitral valve disease, whether MR or mitral stenosis, is currently being studied using various device types and designs. We will discuss these separately under the dedicated TMVR device section.

3. Scientific evidence supporting TMVR

The scientific evidence supporting TMVR is based on observational data, mostly from registries, in North America and Europe [1, 4–15], summarized in **Table 1**. Several studies showed data on outcomes of mitral ViV, ViR, ViMAC from single or multi-center registries; with consistent results demonstrating overall better outcomes for mitral ViV procedures compared to mitral ViR and ViMAC [1, 4–15].

The role of mitral ViV, ViR, and ViMAC has been evaluated in a prospective early feasibility clinical trial, the MITRAL trial (Mitral Implantation of Transcatheter Valves, NCT 02370511), which is the first prospective study assessing outcomes of TMVR in all of the three separate subtypes. The results of the trial have been recently published [16–18].

Author, year published	Number of patients	Major outcomes
Guerrero et al. [11]	64 patients with ViMAC	• Technical success was 72% • 30-day all-cause mortality was 29.7% • 84% of the survivors with follow-up data available were in New York Heart Association (NYHA) class I or II at 30 days
Yoon et al. [13]	248, 176 patients undergoing ViV, 72 patients undergoing ViR	• ViR had lower technical success (83.3% vs. 96.0%; p = 0.001) due to more frequent second valve implantation (11.1% vs. 2.8%; p = 0.008) • ViR had higher 1-year all-cause mortality rate (28.7% vs. 12.6%; log-rank test, p = 0.01).
Eleid et al. [14]	87 patients (ViV = 60, ViR = 15, ViMAC = 12)	• Procedural success was 97% in ViV, and 74% in ViR and ViMAC. • 30-day survival free of death and cardiovascular surgery was 95% in ViV and 78% in ViR and ViMAC • 1-year survival free of death and cardiovascular surgery was 86% in the ViV compared with 68% in ViR and ViMAC
Guerrero et al. [5]	106 patients with MAC	• 30-day and 1-year all-cause mortality was 25% and 53.7%, respectively. • Most patients who survived 30 days were alive at 1 year and majority were in NYHA functional class I or II

Author, year published	Number of patients	Major outcomes
Urena et al. [12]	91 patients (ViV 37.3%, ViR in 33.0%, and ViMAC in 29.7%)	• mortality rate at 30 days was 7.7% without significant differences between groups • The cumulative rates of all-cause mortality at 1-year and 2-year follow-up were 21.0% and 35.7%, respectively, with higher late mortality in patients with MAC.
Yoon et al. [1]	521 patients (322 ViV, 141 ViR, and 58 ViMAC)	• ViMAC was associated with higher all-cause mortality in comparison to ViR and ViV at follow up of 30 days (34.5% vs. 9.9% vs. 6.2%; log-rank $P < 0.001$) and 1 year (62.8% vs. 30.6% vs. 14.0%; log-rank $P < 0.001$).
Werner et al. [15]	7 patients (3 ViV, 1 ViR, 3 ViMAC)	• clinical success with functional improvement of at least one NYHA class was achieved in all patients with in-hospital mortality rate of 14% (1/7) • After hospital discharge, no death occurred, and clinical improvement remained stable at 1 year
Guerrero et al. [4]	903 patients (680 ViV, 123 ViR, 100 ViMAC)	• Technical and procedural success were higher in ViV. • In-hospital mortality (ViV = 6.3%, ViR = 9%, ViMAC = 18%; $P = 0.004$) and 30-day mortality (ViV = 8.1%, ViR = 11.5%, ViMAC = 21.8%; $P = 0.003$) were higher in ViMAC.

Table 1.
Summary of observational TMVR studies with their major outcomes.

In the MITRAL trial, in which 30 patients undergoing transseptal mitral ViV were enrolled between July 2016 and October 2017, technical success was achieved in 100% of cases with 30-day all-cause mortality of 3.3%, which remained unchanged at 1 year. At 1-year follow-up, the vast majority of patients were in New York Heart Association (NYHA) functional class I or II [16].

Similarly, in the MITRAL trial assessing patients undergoing transeptal mitral ViR, 30 patients were studied with results showing technical success of 66.7% (driven primarily by need for a second valve in 6 patients), all-cause mortality of 6.7% at 30 days and 23.3% at 1 year. Similar to ViV study, the vast majority of patients were in NYHA class I or II at 1 year [17].

MITRAL trial assessed ViMAC by prospectively enrolling 31 patients and was challenged by a high proportion of patients with threatened left ventricular outflow tract (LVOT) obstruction. As such mitigation strategies were devise in the form of alcohol septal ablation and trans-atrial valve implantation accompanied by anterior leaflet resection. As such as high proportion of patients received trans-atrial TMVR (48.4%), while transseptal access was used in 48.4%, and transapical access 3.2%. Technical success was achieved in 74.2% of cases, overall 16.7% (trans-atrial, 21.4%; transseptal, 6.7%; transapical, 100% [n 1/4 1]; $p = 0.33$) all-cause mortality rate at 30 days and 34.5% (trans-atrial, 38.5%; transseptal, 26.7%; $p = 0.69$) mortality at 1 year. Similar to ViV and ViR study, the vast majority of patients were in NYHA class I or II at 1 year [18]. Importantly, this trial introduced preemptive alcohol septal ablation as a mitigation strategy to prevent LVOT obstruction [18].

4. Procedural planning

Successful TMVR depends on accurate sizing of the mitral annulus and avoidance of LVOT obstruction. In the absence of a validated standard method for mitral annulus sizing at the present time, operators have extrapolated from transcatheter aortic valve replacement (TAVR) experience and used a variety of sizing approaches including echocardiography, 3-dimensional (3D) transesophageal echocardiography, cardiac CT, and balloon sizing techniques [10]. Cardiac CT is the most accepted imaging modality for annulus sizing. In general, pre-procedural imaging constitutes of contrast-enhanced CT to identify critical cardiac structures and anatomy, including sizing of the mitral annulus, which is the basal-most structure of the mitral leaflets [19]. In addition to annular sizing, CT also provides essential information for pre-procedural planning, including the amount and distribution of calcifications, as well as predictors of LVOT obstruction; the left ventricular cavity size, anterior leaflet length, aorto-mitral angulation, septal hypertrophy, among other features. CT is also helpful in identifying the trajectory and site of access, whether transapical or transseptal [10, 19].

Data utilizing 2-dimensional (2D) echo imaging correlated acute angulation of the mitral aorta-outflow-angle (mAOA) with higher risk of LVOT obstruction compared with that of more obtuse mAOA. However, risk of LVOT obstruction is not solely based on mAOA; this is because LVOT is a 3D anatomical structure and mAOA on 2D echo images may not provide the comprehensive assessment needed. CT overcomes this limitation as it provides a 3D assessment. Both the prosthetic valve and the anterior displacement of anterior mitral leaflet can result in severe LVOT obstruction. Additionally, utilization of computer-aided designs and 3-D printed models allows us to test devices in patient-specific anatomy and at different angulations and depths with estimation of risk for LVOT obstruction [19].

LVOT obstruction is a fatal complication; thus, pre-procedural planning in an attempt to predict neo-LVOT provides a key step in the success of TMVR procedure. In a multicenter study of 38 patients undergoing TMVR using balloon-expandable valves for severe mitral valve dysfunction because of degenerative surgical mitral ring, bio-prosthesis, or severe native mitral stenosis from severe mitral annular calcification, the investigators defined LVOT obstruction as increase of 10 mmHg or more in LVOT peak gradient following TMVR and found that 7 of the 38 patients had LVOT obstruction, with CT neo-LVOT surface area correlating well with measurements after TMVR [20]. Yoon and colleagues in their study of 194 patients undergoing TMVR found that LVOT obstruction was associated with higher procedural mortality compared with patients without LVOT obstruction (34.6% vs. 2.4%; $p < 0.001$) [21].

5. Technical considerations

The first few TMVR procedures were performed using a surgical transapical [6, 7] or open trans-atrial [8, 9] approach, but subsequent reports described successful implantation with a completely percutaneous trans-femoral transseptal approach [10–12]. Transseptal access has been the default access in ViV and ViR in the MITRAL trial, while both transseptal and trans-atrial access have been equally used in ViMAC [16–18]. All-cause 30-day mortality in ViMAC was 16.7% (trans-atrial, 21.4%; transseptal, 6.7%; transapical, 100% [n = 1]; p 0.33) and 1-year mortality was 34.5% (trans-atrial, 38.5%; transseptal, 26.7%; p = 0.69) [18]. These mortality rates are relatively higher than other transeptal or transapical procedures; as studies have shown that the 30-day and 1-year mortality rates were 3.6% and 23.2% for patients undergoing transseptal transcatheter edge-to-edge repair using MitraClip for secondary mitral regurgitation, and the 30-day and 1-year mortality rates were 8.4% and 25.4% for transapical TAVR [22, 23].

Because the mitral annulus is larger in size compared to aortic valve annulus, TMVR requires larger devices, including prosthesis and delivery systems [10]. Mitral annular calcifications are less common compared with aortic valve calcifications, and their presence may condition the implant of a transcatheter mitral prosthesis. For this purpose, the role of TMVR in presence of considerable annular calcification is less clear, as shown in the MAC (mitral annular calcification) Global Registry, which demonstrated that TMVR was feasible in MAC but associated with relatively high early and midterm mortality at 1 year, although patients who survived at 1-year follow-up had sustained improvement of symptoms [4, 5]. Similarly, the MITRAL trial showed relatively high 1-year mortality in ViMAC patients, but transeptal ViMAC showed promising results with 30-day mortality lower than the predicted STS score, however mortality rates in this population remains higher than other transeptal procedures, including transcatheter edge-to-edge repair using MitraClip [1, 2, 18].

6. Procedural complications

6.1 ViV

Complications in ViV are considered relatively low, with reported LV perforation 0.4%, LVOT obstruction 0.7% and conversion to surgery in 1.3% [1, 4]. Post-procedure mitral valve function was excellent with a median mean mitral valve gradient of 4 mm Hg and residual mitral regurgitation grade of 1+ or less in 98.1%. A second valve was needed in a relatively small proportion of mitral ViV patients (1.5%) and was associated with higher mortality at 30 days. The reasons or mechanisms for which this was associated with higher mortality (residual mitral regurgitation, thrombosis, renal failure) are not known at this time [4].

6.2 VIR

Generally speaking, studies have shown that ViR TMVR is associated with worse outcomes compared with ViV, but better outcomes compared with ViMAC procedures [1, 4, 10, 16–18]; ViR is a more complex procedure than ViV due to the different types of rings (rigid versus nonrigid, complete versus incomplete) and different shapes, which are usually not round predisposing to residual paravalvular leak [1, 4]. There are 3 main challenges in ViR cases: valve anchoring, LVOTO and paravalvular leak. Yoon et al. showed that ViR had a significantly lower technical success rate compared with the ViV group (83.3% vs. 96.0%; p = 0.001) due to more frequent second valve implantation (11.1% vs. 2.8%; p = 0.008) [1]. Moreover, the investigators found that residual mitral regurgitation moderate or higher at 30 days was more frequent in patients with flexible rings compared with those with semi-rigid rings (44.4% vs. 10.8%, p = 0.02) [1]. A study showed that the 30-day mortality was 11.5% in ViR patients with median STS PROM score of 9.3% [4]. The reasons for higher mortality in mitral ViR are probably multifactorial; potentially related to higher procedural complication rates including LVOT obstruction, higher valve embolization rate, residual mitral regurgitation and need for reintervention including conversion to surgery, as well as different baseline characteristics including a lower baseline left ventricular ejection fraction [4]. In fact, the ViR group also had the highest rate of device embolization at 30 days 3.6% compared with mitral ViV 0.2% and ViMAC 1.6% [4].

Guerrero et al. showed 4.9% rate of LVOT obstruction in ViR, which was lower than the 8% in the VIVID registry; this could be related to increased experience in patient selection and risk-reduction strategies. Overall, mitral ViR is observed to have higher rates of LVOTO as compared to ViV, possibly due to the presence of a preserved anterior mitral leaflet. In most ViV cases, the anterior leaflet is no longer present making LVOT obstruction less likely [4].

Guerrero et al. also demonstrated that when comparing outcomes by types of rings (complete versus incomplete, rigid versus nonrigid), there was a larger mitral valve area in incomplete rings versus complete rings [4]. However, there was no statistically significant difference in median mean mitral valve gradients and clinical outcomes between the groups based on the type of ring [4].

6.3 ViMAC

Studies have shown that ViMAC procedures were associated with the lowest technical success and the highest in-hospital and 30-mortality compared with mitral ViR and ViV [1, 4]. Similar to ViR, ViMAC has significant challenges to anchoring, paravalvular leak and LVOTO. The reasons are multifactorial, including presence of multiple comorbidities and technical challenges including the complexity of the mitral valve anatomy; as the native mitral valve is a saddle oval shape being treated with a round transcatheter valve which may lead to paravalvular leak at commissures, non-uniform calcium distribution, and relatively small sized ventricles accompanied by threatened LVOTO [1, 4, 10]. Therefore, there is a frequent need for LVOT modification taking the form of three options: LAMPOON, Alcohol septal ablations or surgical resection of the anterior leaflet.

LVOT obstruction is considered the Achilles' heel of TMVR, especially in ViMAC. It has limited treatment options and was the strongest predictor of 30-day and 1-year mortality in the TMVR in MAC Global Registry [4, 5, 10]. Studies have shown that LVOT obstruction rate in ViMAC procedures is at least 10% [1, 4, 5, 10]. One factor that could contribute to different rates of LVOT obstruction observed among registries may be the different definitions used, such as LVOT obstruction with hemodynamic compromise versus increase in mean LVOT gradient of ≥10 mm Hg from baseline. Another important factor may be improved screening process with cardiac computed tomography to predict LVOT obstruction and strategies to prevent it [1, 4]. Potential predictors of LVOT obstruction are the angle of the mitral valve in relation to the LVOT long axis, the presence of small LV cavity, bulging or severe hypertrophy of the basal interventricular septum, long anterior mitral valve leaflets, dynamic alterations as the pushing of the native anterior leaflet toward the LVOT, prosthesis protrusion and device flaring [4, 5, 10, 19–21].

7. Strategies to mitigate procedural complications

Cardiac computed tomography to measure the expected neo-LVOT area to assess the risk of TMVR-induced LVOT obstruction identifying patients at risk facilitates implementation of measures to decrease such risk including preemptive alcohol septal ablation, percutaneous laceration of the anterior mitral leaflet, surgical excision of the anterior mitral leaflet during trans-atrial TMVR or deciding not to perform the procedure at all [1, 4, 10, 24, 25].

Several strategies to prevent or treat LVOT obstruction caused by TMVR have been developed and studied. These strategies include: 1) preemptive alcohol septal ablation in patients at risk for TMVR-induced LVOT obstruction who have favorable anatomy for alcohol ablation as shown in the MITRAL trial [18], 2) percutaneous laceration of the anterior leaflet to decrease the risk of TMVR-induced LVOT obstruction in TMVR procedures (The LAMPOON trial; Laceration of the Anterior Mitral Leaflet to Prevent Outflow Obstruction During TMVR) [24, 25], 3) possibly trans-atrial surgical access for TMVR in severe MAC, as evaluated by the SITRAL Trial (Surgical Implantation of Transcatheter Valves) [1, 4, 24, 25].

8. Dedicated TMVR devices

In addition to the balloon expandable valves which were initially designed for the aortic valve and have been used in mitral valve interventions, several valve designs dedicated to the mitral valve have been developed and studied in several studies with a relatively small number of patients, with some promising results [10]. These dedicated mitral valves are summarized in **Figure 1** and **Table 2**.

The CardiAQ (Edwards Lifesciences Inc) valve is a nitinol self-expanding tri-leaflet valve, composed of bovine pericardial tissue, which was the first dedicated device for TMVR in 2012 in high-risk patients with severe MR. This was followed by the second generation of the valve, which was used for the first time in 2014 [26]. The new redesigned version was renamed as the EVOQUE valve. It offers both a transapical and transfemoral-transseptal approach. The EVOQUE valve offered enhanced maneuverability and depth control, and lower ventricular projection to avoid LVOT obstruction. Currently, the Edwards EVOQUE TMVR Early Feasibility Study (NCT02718001) is recruiting and will assess feasibility at 30 days. The RELIEF (Reduction or Elimination of Mitral Regurgitation in Degenerative or Functional Mitral Regurgitation With the CardiAQ-Edwards™ Transcatheter Mitral Valve, NCT02722551) trial was stopped by the Edwards Company for further design validation. From the preliminary results presented, 13 patients have been treated with technical success of 92% and high mortality rate of 45% at 30 days [10, 27].

The Tiara (Neovasc Inc., Canada) valve is a bioprosthetic valve; it constitutes of bovine pericardial tissue, which is mounted inside a nitinol frame. It is self-expanding and has a relatively large atrial skirt, which decreases the risk of paravalvular leaks. The first implant of Tiara valve was performed in Vancouver in 2014. The two major studies of the Tiara valves, TIARA-I (Early Feasibility Study of the

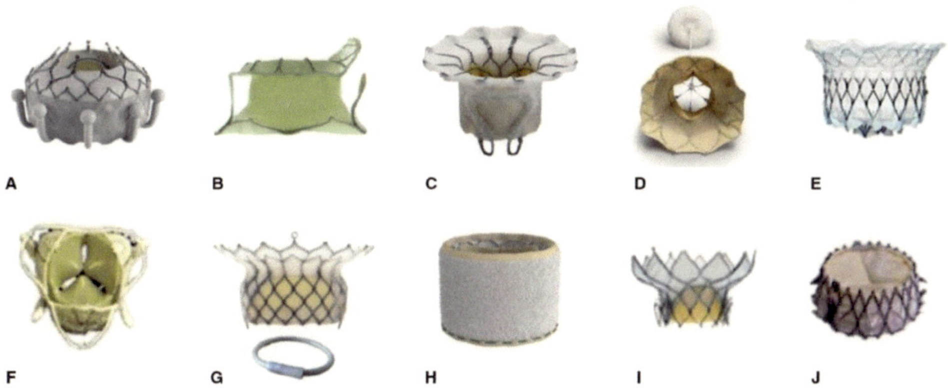

Figure 1.
Current transcatheter mitral valve replacement devices. **A,** *CardiAQ/EVOQUE (Edwards Lifesciences Inc).* **B,** *Tiara (Neovasc Inc., Canada).* **C,** *FORTIS (Edwards Lifesciences Inc).* **D,** *Tendyne (Abbott Inc).* **E,** *intrepid (Medtronic Inc).* **F,** *caisson (LivaNova, UK).* **G,** *HighLife bioprosthesis and sub-annular implant (HighLife SAS, France).* **H,** *SAPIEN M3 (Edwards Lifesciences Inc).* **I,** *Cardiovalve (Cardiovalve, Israel).* **J,** *Navi-gate (NaviGate cardiac structures, Inc., CA). Obtained with permission from Testa et al. publication [10].*

Device name	Brief description	Number of patients	Primary outcomes
CardiAQ-EVOQUE (Edwards Lifesciences Inc)	• Nitinol self-expanding tri-leaflet valve, composed of bovine pericardial tissue • Transapical/transseptal • EVOQUE valve: new redesigned version of the valve	13	Technical success, 92% Mortality at 30 days, 45%
Tiara (Neovasc Inc., Canada)	• Nitinol self-expanding tri-leaflet valve of bovine pericardial tissue • Transapical	30	Technical success, 90% Mortality at 30 d, 10%
FORTIS (Edwards Lifesciences Inc)	• Nitinol self-expanding tri-leaflet valve of bovine pericardial tissue • Transapical	13	Technical success, 76.9% Mortality at 30 d, 38.5%
Tendyne (Abbott Inc)	• Self-expanding tri-leaflet valve of porcine pericardial tissue, mounted on nitinol double-frame stent • Transapical	100	Technical success, 96% Mortality at 30 d, 6%
Intrepid (Medtronic Inc)	• Nitinol self-expanding tri-leaflet valve of bovine pericardial tissue • Transapical (transseptal approach under development)	50	Technical success, 96% Mortality at 30 d, 14%
Caisson (LivaNova, UK)	• Nitinol self-expanding tri-leaflet valve of porcine pericardial tissue, with a D-shaped anchor • Transseptal	NA	NA
HighLife (HighLife SAS, France)	• Two separate components: nitinol alloy-based self-expanding frame with a tri-leaflet valve of bovine pericardium tissue and a sub-annular implant • Transapical/trans-atrial (transseptal approach under development)	Anecdotal cases	Promising results in anecdotal cases
SAPIEN M3 (Edwards Lifesciences Inc)	• Nitinol docking system and a modified SAPIEN 3 valve • Transseptal	15	Technical success, 86.7% Mortality at 30 d, 0%
Cardiovalve (Cardiovalve, Israel)	• Dual nitinol frame with a tri-leaflet bovine pericardium valve • Transseptal	5	Technical success, 100% Mortality at 30 d, 60%
Cephea (Cephea Valve Technologies)	• Self-expanding double-disk and tri-leaflet bovine pericardium tissue • Transseptal/trans-atrial	Preclinical models First-in-human cases	Promising results in reported cases
AltaValve (4C Medical Technologies Inc)	• Self-expanding supra-annular device, with a bovine tissue valve mounted into a spherical nitinol frame • Transapical	Preclinical models Anecdotal first-in-human case (n = 1)	Promising results in models and reported case

Device name	Brief description	Number of patients	Primary outcomes
NaviGate (NaviGate Cardiac Structures Inc)	• Nitinol self-expandable system with several annular winglets • Transapical	Case report	Promising result in reported cases.

Table 2.
Summary of dedicated TAMR devices and primary outcomes of available early feasibility studies.

Neovasc Tiara Mitral Valve System) (NCT02276547) and the latest TIARA-II (Tiara Transcatheter Mitral Valve Replacement Study), are actively enrolling patients, with promising preliminary results in 71 patients, mostly in functional MR (61%), showing 94% technical success rate, with a mortality rate of 11.3% at 30 days [28, 29].

The FORTIS (Edwards Lifesciences Inc) valve is a self-expanding bioprosthetic valve of bovine pericardial tissue. The first FORTIS implant was performed in 2014. Preliminary results demonstrated outcomes of 13 patients with procedural success of 76.9%. In the early experience, the study was put on hold due to reported valve thrombosis [30].

The Tendyne MV system (Abbott Inc) is a self-expanding porcine pericardial valve, which is mounted on a nitinol stent. It is implanted using the transapical approach and the device is anchored to the annulus using apical tethers. The first Tendyne MV implant was performed in 2014. The Feasibility Study of the Tendyne Mitral Valve System for Use in Subjects With Mitral Annular Calcification (NCT03539458) of the first 100 patients showed that the technical success rate was 97% with no periprocedural mortality and 30-day mortality rate of 6% [31]. Most patients (98.8%) had non-significant MR at 30 days [31]. Importantly, the SUMMIT (Clinical Trial to Evaluate the Safety and Effectiveness of Using the Tendyne Mitral Valve System for the Treatment of Symptomatic Mitral Regurgitation; NCT03433274) is an ongoing multi-center clinical trial randomizing patients to TMVR using the Tendyne valve versus conventional mitral valve surgery, with goal to enroll 1010 patients and expected completion year in 2026.

The Intrepid (Medtronic Inc) valve is a bovine pericardial valve fixed onto a self-expanding nitinol frame. The valve is implanted via transapical access in the majority of cases, but a transseptal approach is being developed. The first implant was performed in 2014. An initial pilot study enrolled 50 high-risk patients with MR and reported 96% success rate, 14% 30-day mortality rate and trivial-trace or mild residual MR at 30 days in all patients [32]. The multicenter randomized APOLLO (Transcatheter Mitral Valve Replacement With the Medtronic Intrepid TMVR System in Patients With Severe Symptomatic Mitral Regurgitation; NCT03242642) trial is still ongoing with patients randomized in a 1:1 fashion to the Intrepid valve versus conventional mitral valve surgery. Outcomes will be evaluated at 30 days, 6 months, and 1 year, with up to 5 years follow-up duration, and estimated study completion date in 2025 [10].

The HighLife (HighLife SAS, France) valve is a 2-component system. The prosthetic valve is implanted in the mitral position and has an anchoring system placed by the trans-arterial retrograde approach in the sub-annular position [10]. Anecdotal initial cases are reported showing acceptable results of the valve [33]. A feasibility trial (NCT02974881) is still active.

The SAPIEN M3 (Edwards Lifesciences Inc) valve is a modified SAPIEN 3 valve. It is implanted using the transseptal approach. It uses nitinol docking system, which allows anchoring of device [10]. From the initial results of feasibility study in 15 patients, technical success was achieved in 86.7%, MR reduction was achieved in

93.3% and no mortality was reported at 30 days [34]. The ENCIRCLE trial is an ongoing study designed to assess the outcomes of the SAPIEN M3 device in 400 patients (NCT04153292).

The Cardiovalve (Cardiovalve, Israel) valve is a bovine pericardial valve mounted on dual nitinol. It is usually implanted using the transseptal approach. The system allows multi-steerable catheter utilization, which provides better control of the device [10]. The AHEAD (European Feasibility Study of the Cardiovalve Transfemoral Mitral Valve System; NCT03339115) study is designed to assess the outcomes of Cardiovalve system in MR. The first 5 cases showed 100% of technical success with significant reduction of MR and absent or non-significant paravalvular leak [35].

The Cephea (Cephea Valve Technologies) system is a repositionable and recapturable frame valve and usually implanted using the transseptal approach. The frame structure allows adequate anchoring independent of the sub-valvular structures. The valve was tested in preclinical models with good performance at 90 days [36]. In addition, early experience with the Cephea device has been reported in 3 patients after the first in-human case with 100% technical success [37, 38]. After a median 6-month follow-up, valve function, echocardiographic parameters and patients' functional status were all favorable [38].

The AltaValve (4C Medical Technologies Inc) is a supra-annular device, which constitutes of bovine tissue mounted onto a nitinol frame. It is a self-expanding valve and implanted using the transseptal or transapical approach. Animal studies showed good performance, and a first-in-human case was performed in Canada in 2018, with satisfactory results [10, 39].

The NaviGate (NaviGate Cardiac Structures Inc) valve is a self-expanding valve and constitutes of a nitinol stent frame and multiple annular winglets, to allow anchoring of the device in the mitral annular position. The valve is implanted using transapical approach. The first in-human valve implant was performed in 2015 in Chile [40]. After an initial interest of this valve in mitral valve position, the device was implanted in the tricuspid position for tricuspid regurgitation using transcatheter interventions with trans-jugular or trans-atrial approach [41].

9. Knowledge gaps and ideas for future research

With the recent advances in TMVR in the most recent years, there remain knowledge gaps and challenges in order to understand the disease and correlate clinical outcomes with this evolving technology. MR is often coexistent with other comorbidities, including valvular disease, such as tricuspid regurgitation, severe pulmonary hypertension, and atrial fibrillation, with significant and independent morbidity and mortality rates [4]. The role of these co-existing factors in this setting is not well-known and should be evaluated in future research.

Studies have shown that TMVR is associated with higher rates of paravalvular leak compared to TAVR; this could be attributed to reduced anatomical support, asymmetrical annulus or asymmetric leaflets in mitral valve compared to aortic valve [4, 10]. Additionally, post-dilation of mitral prosthetic valve could potentially be challenging and risky; due to the close proximity of the mitral valve to the left circumflex artery, the conduction system and the aortic valve. In addition, efforts to avoid damage to sub-valvular structures should be pursued [4, 10]. Future improvement of the dedicated TMVR-specific device design should address these anatomical issues. As we discussed in the previous section, different transcatheter devices have been designed for the treatment of MR (and, in some cases, for off-label treatment of mitral stenosis). Most of the TMVR technologies are still under clinical investigation. Thus, data about their rates of structural deterioration and durability is limited [10].

At the present time, clinical outcomes we have are based on data of mainly the first and second generation prosthetic valves. Outcomes may potentially improve with newer generation devices, improvement in the process of patient selection, operators' experience and innovations in procedural techniques [4]. Newer generation valves with repositionable and retrievable ability could be of benefit in certain patients. For example, the Lotus valve (Boston Scientific, Marlborough, Massachusetts) and Direct Flow (Direct Flow Medical Inc. Santa Rosa, California) valves have been successfully implanted in patients with severe MAC, however the outcomes of these valves should be assessed in future randomized clinical trials utilizing larger number of patients [11].

In conclusion, we have seen several advances in TMVR in the past decade with promising results. However, there remain challenges that need to be evaluated in future studies in order to optimize our procedural success, device evolution, and clinical outcomes to make this new cutting-edge technology available for high-risk patients.

Author details

Lina Ya'qoub* and Marvin Eng
Henry Ford Hospital, Detroit, MI, USA

*Address all correspondence to: yaqoublina1989@gmail.com

References

[1] Yoon SH, Whisenant BK, Bleiziffer S, Delgado V, Dhoble A, Schofer N, Eschenbach L, Bansal E, Murdoch DJ, Ancona Met al.. Outcomes of transcatheter mitral valve replacement for degenerated bioprostheses, failed annuloplasty rings, and mitral annular calcification.**Eur Heart J**. 2019; 40:441-451. doi: 10.1093/eurheartj/ehy590. https://pubmed.ncbi.nlm.nih.gov/30357365/

[2] Jamieson WR, Burr LH, Miyagishima RT, Janusz MT, Fradet GJ, Lichtenstein SV, Ling H. Reoperation for bioprosthetic mitral structural failure: risk assessment. Circulation. 2003 Sep 9;108 Suppl 1:II98-102. doi: 10.1161/01.cir.0000089184.46999.f4. PMID: 12970216.

[3] Expósito V, García-Camarero T, Bernal JM, Arnáiz E, Sarralde A, García I, Berrazueta JR, Revuelta JM. Repeat mitral valve replacement: 30-years' experience.**Rev Esp Cardiol**. 2009; 62:929-932. doi: 10.1016/s1885-5857(09)72658-1

[4] Guerrero M, Vemulapalli S, Xiang Q, Wang DD, Eleid M, Cabalka AK, Sandhu G, Salinger M, Russell H, Greenbaum A, Kodali S, George I, Dvir D, Whisenant B, Russo MJ, Pershad A, Fang K, Coylewright M, Shah P, Babaliaros V, Khan JM, Tommaso C, Saucedo J, Kar S, Makkar R, Mack M, Holmes D, Leon M, Bapat V, Thourani VH, Rihal C, O'Neill W, Feldman T. Thirty-Day Outcomes of Transcatheter Mitral Valve Replacement for Degenerated Mitral Bioprostheses (Valve-in-Valve), Failed Surgical Rings (Valve-in-Ring), and Native Valve With Severe Mitral Annular Calcification (Valve-in-Mitral Annular Calcification) in the United States: Data From the Society of Thoracic Surgeons/American College of Cardiology/Transcatheter Valve Therapy Registry. Circ Cardiovasc Interv. 2020 Mar;13(3):e008425. doi: 10.1161/CIRCINTERVENTIONS.119.008425. Epub 2020 Mar 6. PMID: 32138529. https://www.ahajournals.org/doi/full/10.1161/CIRCINTERVENTIONS.119.008425

[5] Guerrero M, Urena M, Himbert D, Wang DD, Eleid M, Kodali S, George I, Chakravarty T, Mathur M, Holzhey D, Pershad A, Fang HK, O'Hair D, Jones N, Mahadevan VS, Dumonteil N, Rodés-Cabau J, Piazza N, Ferrari E, Ciaburri D, Nejjari M, DeLago A, Sorajja P, Zahr F, Rajagopal V, Whisenant B, Shah PB, Sinning JM, Witkowski A, Eltchaninoff H, Dvir D, Martin B, Attizzani GF, Gaia D, Nunes NSV, Fassa AA, Kerendi F, Pavlides G, Iyer V, Kaddissi G, Witzke C, Wudel J, Mishkel G, Raybuck B, Wang C, Waksman R, Palacios I, Cribier A, Webb J, Bapat V, Reisman M, Makkar R, Leon M, Rihal C, Vahanian A, O'Neill W, Feldman T. 1-Year Outcomes of Transcatheter Mitral Valve Replacement in Patients With Severe Mitral Annular Calcification. J Am Coll Cardiol. 2018 May 1;71(17):1841-1853. doi: 10.1016/j.jacc.2018.02.054. PMID: 29699609. https://www.sciencedirect.com/science/article/abs/pii/S0735109718334934?via%3Dihub

[6] Hasan R, Mahadevan VS, Schneider H, Clarke B. First in human transapical implantation of an inverted transcatheter aortic valve prosthesis totreat native mitral valve stenosis. Circulation 2013;128:e74-6.

[7] Sinning JM, Mellert F, Schiller W, Welz A, Nickenig G, Hammerstingl C. Transcatheter mitral valve replacement using a balloon-expandable prosthesis in a patient with calcified native mitral valve stenosis. Eur Heart J 2013;34:2609.

[8] Wilbring M, Alexiou K, Tugtekin SM, et al. Pushing the limits—further evolutions of trans-catheter valve procedures in the mitral position, including valve-in-valve, valve-in-ring, and valve-in-native-ring. J Thorac Cardiovasc Surg 2014;147:210-9.

[9] Ferrari E, Niclauss L, Locca D, Marcucci C. On-pump fibrillating heart mitral valve replacement with the SAPIEN XT transcatheter heart valve. Eur J Cardiothorac Surg 2014;45:749-51.

[10] Testa L, Popolo Rubbio A, Casenghi M, Pero G, Latib A, Bedogni F. Transcatheter Mitral Valve Replacement in the Transcatheter Aortic Valve Replacement Era. J Am Heart Assoc. 2019 Nov 19;8(22):e013352. doi: 10.1161/JAHA.119.013352. Epub 2019 Nov 7. PMID: 31694451; PMCID: PMC6915270. https://www.ahajournals.org/doi/full/10.1161/JAHA.119.013352

[11] Guerrero M, Dvir D, Himbert D, Urena M, Eleid M, Wang DD, Greenbaum A, Mahadevan VS, Holzhey D, O'Hair D, Dumonteil N, Rodés-Cabau J, Piazza N, Palma JH, DeLago A, Ferrari E, Witkowski A, Wendler O, Kornowski R, Martinez-Clark P, Ciaburri D, Shemin R, Alnasser S, McAllister D, Bena M, Kerendi F, Pavlides G, Sobrinho JJ, Attizzani GF, George I, Nickenig G, Fassa AA, Cribier A, Bapat V, Feldman T, Rihal C, Vahanian A, Webb J, O'Neill W. Transcatheter Mitral Valve Replacement in Native Mitral Valve Disease With Severe Mitral Annular Calcification: Results From the First Multicenter Global Registry. JACC Cardiovasc Interv. 2016 Jul 11;9(13):1361-71. doi: 10.1016/j.jcin.2016.04.022. PMID: 27388824. https://www.sciencedirect.com/science/article/pii/S1936879816304575

[12] Urena M, Brochet E, Lecomte M, Kerneis C, Carrasco JL, Ghodbane W, Abtan J, Alkhoder S, Raffoul R, Iung B, et al.. Clinical and haemodynamic outcomes of balloon-expandable transcatheter mitral valve implantation: a 7-year experience.**Eur Heart J**. 2018; 39:2679-2689. doi: 10.1093/eurheartj/ehy271. https://pubmed.ncbi.nlm.nih.gov/29788044/

[13] Yoon SH, Whisenant BK, Bleiziffer S, Delgado V, Schofer N, Eschenbach L, Fujita B, Sharma R, Ancona M, Yzeiraj Eet al.. Transcatheter mitral valve replacement for degenerated bioprosthetic valves and failed annuloplasty rings.**J Am Coll Cardiol**. 2017; 70:1121-1131. doi: 10.1016/j.jacc.2017.07. https://pubmed.ncbi.nlm.nih.gov/28838360/

[14] Eleid MF, Whisenant BK, Cabalka AK, Williams MR, Nejjari M, Attias D, Fam N, Amoroso N, Foley TA, Pollak PMet al.. Early outcomes of percutaneous transvenous transseptal transcatheter valve implantation in failed bioprosthetic mitral valves, ring annuloplasty, and severe mitral annular calcification.**JACC Cardiovasc Interv**. 2017; 10:1932-1942. doi: 10.1016/j.jcin.2017.08.014. https://pubmed.ncbi.nlm.nih.gov/28982556/

[15] Werner N, Kilkowski C, Sutor D, Weisse U, Schneider S, Zahn R. Transcatheter Mitral Valve Implantation (TMVI) Using Edwards SAPIEN 3 Prostheses in Patients at Very High or Prohibitive Surgical Risk: A Single-Center Experience. J Interv Cardiol. 2020 Jan 6;2020:9485247. doi: 10.1155/2020/9485247. PMID: 31992963; PMCID: PMC6973192. https://www.hindawi.com/journals/jitc/2020/9485247/

[16] Guerrero M, Pursnani A, Narang A, Salinger M, Wang DD, Eleid M, Kodali SK, George I, Satler L, Waksman R, Meduri CU, Rajagopal V, Inglessis I, Palacios I, Reisman M, Eng MH, Russell HM, Pershad A, Fang K, Kar S, Makkar R, Saucedo J, Pearson P, Bokhary U, Kaptzan T, Lewis B, Tommaso C, Krause P,

Thaden J, Oh J, Lang RM, Hahn RT, Leon MB, O'Neill WW, Feldman T, Rihal C. Prospective Evaluation of Transseptal TMVR for Failed Surgical Bioprostheses: MITRAL Trial Valve-in-Valve Arm 1-Year Outcomes. JACC Cardiovasc Interv. 2021 Apr 26;14(8):859-872. doi: 10.1016/j.jcin.2021.02.027. PMID: 33888231.

[17] Guerrero M, Wang DD, Pursnani A, Salinger M, Russell HM, Eleid M, Chakravarty T, Ng MH, Kodali SK, Meduri CU, Pershad A, Satler L, Waksman R, Palacios I, Smalling R, Reisman M, Gegenhuber M, Kaptzan T, Lewis B, Tommaso C, Krause P, Thaden J, Oh J, Douglas PS, Hahn RT, Kar S, Makkar R, Leon MB, Feldman T, Rihal C, O'Neill WW. Prospective Evaluation of TMVR for Failed Surgical Annuloplasty Rings: MITRAL Trial Valve-in-Ring Arm 1-Year Outcomes. JACC Cardiovasc Interv. 2021 Apr 26;14(8):846-858. doi: 10.1016/j.jcin.2021.01.051. PMID: 33888230.

[18] Guerrero M, Wang DD, Eleid MF, Pursnani A, Salinger M, Russell HM, Kodali SK, George I, Bapat VN, Dangas GD, Tang GHL, Inglesis I, Meduri CU, Palacios I, Reisman M, Whisenant BK, Jermihov A, Kaptzan T, Lewis BR, Tommaso C, Krause P, Thaden J, Oh JK, Douglas PS, Hahn RT, Leon MB, Rihal CS, Feldman T, O'Neill WW. Prospective Study of TMVR Using Balloon-Expandable Aortic Transcatheter Valves in MAC: MITRAL Trial 1-Year Outcomes. JACC Cardiovasc Interv. 2021 Apr 26;14(8):830-845. doi: 10.1016/j.jcin.2021.01.052. PMID: 33888229.

[19] Wang DD, Eng M, Greenbaum A, Myers E, Forbes M, Pantelic M, Song T, Nelson C, Divine G, Taylor Aet al.. Predicting LVOT obstruction after TMVR.**JACC Cardiovasc Imaging**. 2016; 9:1349-1352. doi: 10.1016/j.jcmg.2016.01.017

[20] Wang DD, Eng MH, Greenbaum AB, Myers E, Forbes M, Karabon P, Pantelic M, Song T, Nadig J, Guerrero Met al.. Validating a prediction modeling tool for left ventricular outflow tract (LVOT) obstruction after transcatheter mitral valve replacement (TMVR).**Catheter Cardiovasc Interv**. 2018; 92:379-387. doi: 10.1002/ccd.27447

[21] Yoon SH, Bleiziffer S, Latib A, Eschenbach L, Ancona M, Vincent F, Kim WK, Unbehaum A, Asami M, Dhoble A, Silaschi M, Frangieh AH, Veulemans V, Tang GHL, Kuwata S, Rampat R, Schmidt T, Patel AJ, Nicz PFG, Nombela-Franco L, Kini A, Kitamura M, Sharma R, Chakravarty T, Hildick-Smith D, Arnold M, de Brito FS Jr, Jensen C, Jung C, Jilaihawi H, Smalling RW, Maisano F, Kasel AM, Treede H, Kempfert J, Pilgrim T, Kar S, Bapat V, Whisenant BK, Van Belle E, Delgado V, Modine T, Bax JJ, Makkar RR. Predictors of Left Ventricular Outflow Tract Obstruction After Transcatheter Mitral Valve Replacement. JACC Cardiovasc Interv. 2019 Jan 28;12(2):182-193. doi: 10.1016/j.jcin.2018.12.001. PMID: 30678797.

[22] Ailawadi G, Lim DS, Mack MJ, Trento A, Kar S, Grayburn PA, Glower DD, Wang A, Foster E, Qasim A, Weissman NJ, Ellis J, Crosson L, Fan F, Kron IL, Pearson PJ, Feldman T; EVEREST II Investigators. One-Year Outcomes After MitraClip for Functional Mitral Regurgitation. Circulation. 2019 Jan 2;139(1):37-47. doi: 10.1161/CIRCULATIONAHA.117.031733. PMID: 30586701. https://www.ahajournals.org/doi/full/10.1161/CIRCULATIONAHA.117.031733

[23] McNeely C, Zajarias A, Robbs R, Markwell S, Vassileva CM. Transcatheter Aortic Valve Replacement Outcomes in Nonagenarians Stratified by Transfemoral and Transapical Approach. Ann Thorac Surg. 2017 Jun;103(6):1808-1814. doi: 10.1016/j.athoracsur.2017.02.056. Epub 2017 Apr 24. PMID: 28450135.

[24] Khan JM, Rogers T, Schenke WH, Mazal JR, Faranesh AZ, Greenbaum AB, Babaliaros VC, Chen MY, Lederman RJ. Intentional laceration of the anterior mitral valve leaflet to prevent left ventricular outflow tract obstruction during transcatheter mitral valve replacement: Pre-clinical findings.**JACC Cardiovasc Interv**. 2016; 9:1835-1843. doi: 10.1016/j.jcin.2016.06.020

[25] Babaliaros VC, Greenbaum AB, Khan JM, Rogers T, Wang DD, Eng MH, O'Neill WW, Paone G, Thourani VH, Lerakis Set al.. Intentional percutaneous laceration of the anterior mitral leaflet to prevent outflow obstruction during transcatheter mitral valve replacement: first-in-human experience.**JACC Cardiovasc Interv**. 2017; 10:798-809. doi: 10.1016/j.jcin.2017.01.035

[26] Søndergaard L, De Backer O, Franzen OW, Holme SJ, Ihlemann N, Vejlstrup NG, Hansen PB, Quadri A. First-in-human case of transfemoral CardiAQ mitral valve implantation. **Circ Cardiovasc Interv**. 2015; 8:e002135.

[27] Søndergaard L. CardiAQ-Edwards TMVR. Paper presented at: PCR London Valves; September 2016; London, United Kingdom.

[28] Cheung A, Stub D, Moss R, Boone RH, Leipsic J, Verheye S, Banai S, Webb J. Transcatheter mitral valve implantation with Tiara bioprosthesis. **EuroIntervention**. 2014; 10:U115–U119

[29] Cheung A. The TIARA Program: Attributes, Challenges, and Early Clinical Data. TVT 2019; June 2019; Chicago, IL

[30] Regueiro A, Ye J, Fam N, Bapat VN, Dagenais F, Peterson MD, Windecker S, Webb JG, Rodés-Cabau J. 2-Year outcomes after transcatheter mitral valve replacement. **JACC Cardiovasc Interv**. 2017; 10:1671-16

[31] Sorajja P, Moat N, Badhwar V, Walters D, Paone G, Bethea B, Bae R, Dahle G, Mumtaz M, Grayburn P, Kapadia S, Babaliaros V, Guerrero M, Satler L, Thourani V, Bedogni F, Rizik D, Denti P, Dumonteil N, Modine T, Sinhal A, Chuang ML, Popma JJ, Blanke P, Leipsic J, Muller D. Initial feasibility study of a new transcatheter mitral prosthesis: the first 100 patients. **J Am Coll Cardiol**. 2019; 73:1250-1260.

[32] Bapat V, Rajagopal V, Meduri C, Farivar RS, Walton A, Duffy SJ, Gooley R, Almeida A, Reardon MJ, Kleiman NS, Spargias K, Pattakos S, Ng MK, Wilson M, Adams DH, Leon M, Mack MJ, Chenoweth S, Sorajja P. Intrepid global pilot study investigators early experience with new transcatheter mitral valve replacement. **J Am Coll Cardiol**. 2018; 71:12-2

[33] Barbanti M, Piazza N, Mangiafico S, Buithieu J, Bleiziffer S, Ronsivalle G, Scandura S, Giuffrida A, Popolo Rubbio A, Mazzamuto M, Sgroi C, Lange R, Tamburino C. Transcatheter mitral valve implantation using the HighLife system. **JACC Cardiovasc Interv**. 2017; 10:1662-1670

[34] Makkar RR. Transcatheter Mitral Valve Replacement with the SAPIEN M3 System: 30-Day Outcomes - U.S. Early Feasibility Study. TCT 2018; September 2018; San Diego, CA

[35] Maisano F. Cardiovalve: device attributes, implant, procedure and early results. TCT 2018; September 2018; San Diego, CA

[36] Granada JF. Cephea TMVR System: device description, clinical appraisal and development plans. TCT 2018; September 2018; San Diego, CA

[37] Modine T, Vahl TP, Khalique OK, Coisne A, Vincent F, Montaigne D, Godart F, Van Belle E, Granada JF. First-in-Human Implant of the Cephea Transseptal Mitral Valve Replacement

System. Circ Cardiovasc Interv. 2019 Sep;12(9):e008003. doi: 10.1161/CIRCINTERVENTIONS.119.008003. Epub 2019 Sep 12. PMID: 31510775.

[38] Alperi A, Dagenais F, Del Val D, Bernier M, Vahl TP, Khalique OK, Modine T, Granada JF, Rodés-Cabau J. Early Experience With a Novel Transfemoral Mitral Valve Implantation System in Complex Degenerative Mitral Regurgitation. JACC Cardiovasc Interv. 2020 Oct 26;13(20):2427-2437. doi: 10.1016/j.jcin.2020.08.006. PMID: 33069643.

[39] Généreux *P. ALTA* Valve: device attributes, implant procedure, and first-in-human. TCT 2018; September 2018; San Diego, CA

[40] Navia JL, Baeza C, Maluenda G, Kapadia S, Elgharably H, Sadowski J, Bartuś K, Beghi C, Thyagarajan K, Bertwell R, Quijano RC. Transcatheter mitral valve replacement with the NaviGate stent in a preclinical model. **EuroIntervention**. 2017; 13:e1401–e1409.

[41] Navia JL, Kapadia S, Elgharably H, Maluenda G, Bartuś K, Baeza C, Nair RK, Rodés-Cabau J, Beghi C, Quijano RC. Transcatheter tricuspid valve implantation of navigate bioprosthesis in a preclinical model. **JACC Basic Transl Sci**. 2018; 3:67-79.

Chapter 6

Percutaneous Treatment of Tricuspid Regurgitation

Carlos Minguito-Carazo, Tomás Benito-González, Rodrigo Estévez-Loureiro, Carmen Garrote-Coloma, Julio Echarte-Morales, Armando Pérez de Prado and Felipe Fernández-Vázquez

Abstract

Tricuspid valve regurgitation is one of the most common valvular disorders and moderate to severe tricuspid regurgitation is consistently associated to an increased morbidity and mortality. From an etiopathological perspective, tricuspid regurgitation can be classified in primary, due to the organic disease of any of the valve components, or secondary, as a result of tricuspid valve annulus dilatation, adverse right ventricular remodeling and tricuspid valve leaflet tethering. Despite its poor prognosis, most patients with tricuspid insufficiency are managed conservatively and only those with concomitant left heart valvular disease do finally go surgery in the real-world setting. In fact, outcomes of conventional surgery in patients with isolated tricuspid regurgitation are poor and this approach has not proven yet any survival benefit over stand-alone medical therapy. Given this unmet need, new transcatheter techniques have been developed in the last years, including leaflet plication, percutaneous annuloplasty and valve implantation in either the tricuspid position (orthotopic implantation) or in a different position such as the vena cava (heterotopic implantation). These techniques, with promising outcomes, are seen as an interesting alternative to open-heart surgery given the much lower periprocedural risk.

Keywords: percutaneous tricuspid valve repair, transcatheter tricuspid valve replacement, tricuspid valve insufficiency, tricuspid regurgitation, tricuspid valve

1. Introduction

Moderate or severe tricuspid regurgitation (TR) is a common disorder affecting over 1.6 million people in the United States and close to 70 million worldwide [1, 2]. In the vast majority of cases, the underlying mechanism is functional, due to right ventricular (RV) remodeling in patients with left-side heart disease, atrial fibrillation, primary pulmonary hypertension (PH) or RV dysfunction [3]. Although TR has been traditionally considered to be a benign valve disorder in comparison with left valve disease, it is conversely associated to a poorer prognosis. Furthermore, this finding has been consistently reported in different clinical scenarios, even in the absence of PH or right-side heart failure (HF) [4, 5]. However, most patients with significant TR only receive medical treatment and very few undergo invasive surgical approach if no concomitant coronary or left valvular disease is present [6]. Thus, surgical tricuspid valve (TV) repair or replacement in isolated TR is fairly indicated and reported periprocedural mortality can be as high as 20% [7, 8]. Recently, new percutaneous techniques have shown promising results for the treatment of TR and appear as an alternative to conventional surgery in those cases where only conservative management could be offered in the past due to high surgical risk. In this chapter we will review the different devices that are currently available and to date published evidence for these approaches.

2. Tricuspid regurgitation

2.1 Anatomy of the tricuspid valve

The TV is a complex structure composed of three leaflets (septal, anterior and posterior), a fibrous TV annulus (TVA) in which these leaflets are inserted, at least two papillary muscles with multiple tendinous cords and the adjacent atrial and RV myocardium. Despite these general considerations, anatomical interindividual variability is high, and it is not so rare to find four or even five TV leaflets instead of three [9–11]. The anterior leaflet is usually more prominent and extends from the infundibular region to the inferolateral wall. The posterior leaflet is smaller and, in some cases, hypoplastic, and it is inserted along the posterior margin of the TVA from the septum to the inferolateral basal segment. Lastly, the septal leaflet is fixed along the interventricular septum from the infundibulum to the posterior ventricular margin.

The fibrous TVA is not a flat structure but elliptic in shape under normal preloading conditions, with the posterolateral portion at a lower or more apical position and the anteroseptal portion in a higher or more atrial situation. Like the mitral valve annulus, the TVA is dynamic and changes shape and size during the cardiac cycle. TV is the largest and the most apically positioned heart valve, and can measure up to 9 cm^2 in size in healthy subjects.

The subvalvular apparatus is composed of the tendinous cords and the papillary muscles. Usually, there are two different papillary muscles, anterior and posterior, but not infrequently, a third septal papillary muscle can be found. The anterior papillary muscle is the largest of these muscles and gives rise to cords that sustain the anterior and posterior leaflets, while the posterior papillary muscle supports mainly the posterior and the septal leaflets. The septal leaflet is normally directly fixed to the septal ventricular wall by third order tendinous cords, resulting in reduced displacement during the cardiac cycle.

From an interventional perspective, some issues should be highlighted that may pose technical difficulties for an invasive approach [12–14]:

- The TV has a close anatomical relationship with other structures such as the non-coronary sinus of Valsalva (adjacent to the anteroseptal commissure), the atrioventricular node and the bundle of His (along the intramembranous portion of the septum) or the right coronary artery (which runs parallelly to the TVA).

- The distance between the outfall of inferior vena cava, the most frequent access for percutaneous TV intervention, and the TV is small, and this can challenge the achievement of coaxiality with the TV coaptation plane.

- Implantable cardiac devices can be frequently found in patients with TR and, even if not related to the mechanism of TR, right atrial and RV leads can difficult an adequate percutaneous approach.

- The anterior position of the tricuspid valve significantly impairs echocardiographic window by transesophageal echocardiography, which has become the main imaging technique for guiding structural and valve transcatheter interventions.

- Severe RV remodeling and systemic congestion can lead to huge dilatation of TVA and tethering of TV leaflets causing very wide gaps, which can limit reliable TV percutaneous intervention.

2.2 Etiology

Competence of the TV depends on the integrity of all its components (leaflets, TVA and subvalvular apparatus). The dysfunction of any of these structures can cause TR and we can differentiate two types according to the mechanism of the valve insufficiency:

a. Primary (10–20%): due to organic disease affecting mainly the TV leaflets and/or the subvalvular apparatus (**Table 1**). This heterogeneous group includes congenital diseases, systemic and local inflammatory or infiltrative disorders, and traumatic damage of the valve [15].

b. Functional (80–90%): this is by far the most common type of TR and it is secondary to any of the following diseases [16–18]:

    - Left-side HF with either preserve or not preserve left ventricular ejection fraction: ischemic heart disease, hypertension, dilated cardiomyopathy, mitral or aortic valvular disease... leading to increased left atrial pressure and postcapillary PH.

    - Precapillary PH and/or primary RV dysfunction.

    - Atrial fibrillation (AF).

From a physiopathological perspective, all these disorders are closely related to each other and frequently two or more of them can coexist in the same patient. In fact, all of them end in a common pathway characterized by progressive TVA dilatation, RV dilatation and dysfunction, and TV leaflet tethering. These changes increase the TR regurgitation, thus, worsening RV adverse remodeling that further impairs the coaptation gap of TV leaflets [19]. Moreover, systemic congestion and

Congenital	Ebstein anomaly Other corrected or non-corrected CHD
Acquired	Infectious Endocarditis Carcinoid syndrome Rheumatic disease Myxomatous degeneration Endomyocardial fibrosis Traumatism (blunt chest trauma) Iatrogenic (ICD leads, EMD, drugs, radiation, surgery)

Table 1.
Causes of primary tricuspid regurgitation. CHD: congenital heart disease, ICD: implantable cardiac devices; EMB: endomyocardial biopsy.

chronic neuro-hormonal activation also contribute to this self-perpetuating mechanism that, if untreated, conducts to irreversible end-stage right HF.

2.3 Diagnosis

To date, transthoracic echocardiography is the gold standard for diagnosis of TR. Current guidelines highlight the importance of a comprehensive evaluation of the TV in order to improve the quality of the diagnosis, but also, the decision-making process, including [20]:

a. TR severy: qualitative, semi-quantitative and quantitative parameters should support the grading of TR.

b. Etiology: primary vs. functional.

c. Mechanism: TVA dilatation, TV leaflet tethering, organic TV disease.

d. Complementary key information:

- Left heart size, function and valve disease.
- Pulmonary artery pressure (PAP).
- RV size and function: tricuspid annular plane systolic excursion (TAPSE), 2D longitudinal strain, RV-PA coupling).
- Fluid status (size of inferior vena cava).

It should be noted that most of these measurements can be significantly affected by the preload conditions of the patient at the time the study is performed. Therefore, intensive intravenous diuretic therapy should be considered in patients with an over-volume status in order to perform the study in an as close to euvolemic state as possible. In this regard, vena contracta width is becoming one of the most used parameters for TR severy grading given its higher independency from preload conditions. Recently, a 5-degree scheme for grading TR based on the vena contracta and the effective regurgitation orifice area has been suggested pointing out the prognosis addictive significance of massive or torrential TR in patients with huge regurgitant orifices compared to severe TR [21] (**Table 2**). In this regard, patients with massive or torrential TR showed a lower survival, higher cardiovascular mortality and more admissions for heart failure than those with severe TR [22].

Echocardiographic parameter	*Mild*	*Moderate*	*Severe*	*Massive*	*Torrential*
VC (biplane)	<3 mm	3-6.9 mm	7-13 mm	14-20 mm	≥ 21 mm
EROA (PISA)	<20 mm^2	20-39 mm^2	40-59 mm^2	60-79 mm^2	≥ 80 mm^2
3D VCA or quantitative EROA			75-94 mm^2	95-114 mm^2	≥ 115 mm^2

Table 2.
New classification for grading the severity of TR. VC: vena contracta; EROA: effective regurgitant orifice area; 3D VCA: three-dimensional vena contracta área.

In addition, right ventricular systolic function assessment is essential when evaluating TR. This has been traditionally addressed by the TAPSE and the fractional area change (FAC). However, recently the RV free wall longitudinal strain (> −23%) has been proposed as an independent risk factor for all-cause mortality and incremental to TAPSE and FAC [23]. In addition, although 3D- echocardiogram could evaluate accurately the RV ejection fraction, cardiac magnetic resonance is still the gold standard method to assess the RV function and volumes.

Together with the development of new percutaneous techniques, advance imaging of TR is also growing, and this evolution will probably contribute to a better understanding of the anatomy and mechanism of this disease. To date, both, transthoracic and, more specifically, transesophageal echocardiography play a key role in the indication of intervention, the selection of candidates for each percutaneous or surgical technique, and as guidance for transcatheter procedures [24]. In the following years, probably the magnetic resonance imaging and computed tomography will provide further insights in this pathology. Furthermore, we expect that all the advances in the field of TV imaging will help to find the optimal timing for intervention, which nowadays is one of the major challenges of this disease.

2.4 Prognosis

Up to mild TR can be oftenly found in healthy individuals. Moreover, the prevalence of moderate to severe TR has increased in the last years and will probably continue to rise given the expected aging of worldwide population. To date, it is frequently associated with other cardiac disorders and can be found in around 15–40% of patients with AF, HF or severe left-side heart valve disease. The presence of significant TR is associated to an increased mortality in different series and this negative impact on outcomes is related to the severity of the TV insufficiency. In a retrospective study including more than 5000 patients, the survival rates at one year were 92% in patients without TR and 90%, 79% and 64% in those with mild, moderate or severe TR, respectively [25]. Likewise, Chorin et al. analyzed over 33.000 echocardiograms performed in a 5-year period. In this large single center cohort, moderate [HR 1.15, 95% CI 1.02–1.3, p = 0.024] and severe TR (HR 1.43, 95% CI 1.08–1.88, p = 0.011) had a worse prognosis than those with no or minimal TR [26].

Topilsky et al. observed similar findings when analyzed a cohort of 353 patients with isolated TR [27]. They concluded that severe isolated TR was an independent predictor of all-cause mortality and found that an effective regurgitant orifice over 40 mm2 was significantly related to a reduced survival independently of other characteristics. It should be highlighted that adverse prognosis impact of moderate or severe TR has been reported in a wide range of diverse clinical scenarios, such as HF with either preserved or reduced left ventricular ejection fraction, atrial fibrillation without left-side HF or mitral or aortic valve disease. Interestingly, a recent meta-analysis including 70 studies and 32601 patients followed during a mean of over 3 years reported that moderate or severe TR was associated with a two-fold increased mortality risk compared to mild or no TR (RR 1.95, 95% CI 1.75–2.17) [4]. This association remained statistically significant when adjusted for systolic pulmonary artery pressure, RV dysfunction, left ventricular ejection fraction, AF or grade of mitral regurgitation.

2.5 Surgical approach

Several surgical approaches to treat TR have been suggested in the last decades. Among them, TV repair has been related to superior outcomes compared to TV replacement [28]. Furthermore, ring annuloplasty offers a consistent reduction in TR in long-term follow up and is nowadays the first line technique in the TV anatomy is suitable [29].

Despite the increasing prevalence of significant TR and its adverse prognosis impact on survival, evidence to date of clinical benefit of open-heart surgery is scarse. Current guidelines in Europe and USA showed a consensual indication for symptomatic primary TR despite medical therapy and for functional TR in patients undergoing left heart valve disease. However, these recommendations have a C level of evidence.

On the contrary, the indication of TV surgery in patients with isolated functional TR is still controversial. Some aspects should be highlighted regarding this issue. First, functional TR is a heterogeneous group including patients at very different stages of TV disease, PH and RV remodeling/function, which might not benefit from the same therapeutical approach. Second, the evaluation of clinical status and its impairment related to TR is oftenly challenging, especially in elderly patients or those with comorbidities. Third, to date, TV surgery has not proven any benefit in hard outcomes compared to conservative management in this population. In this regard, Axtell et al. assessed outcomes in a retrospective cohort of 3276 patients with isolated TR. In this study, there were no differences in survival between patients who received medical versus surgical therapy (HR: 1.34; 95% CI 0.78–2.30; p = 0.288). And four, reported outcomes of isolated TV surgery are poor. Alqahtani et al. recently reviewed trends and outcomes of isolated TV surgery in USA during over a decade [8]. They concluded that isolated repair was associated with high in-hospital mortality (8.1%) and significant rates of permanent pacemaker implantation (10.9%) and new dialysis (4.4%). Morbidity and mortality were even worse among those patients who underwent TV replacement (10.9%, 34.1% and 5.5%, respectively). Similarly, Dreyfus reported an in-hospital mortality of 10% and 19% of major complications during admission in a series of 241 patients who underwent isolated TV surgery in France during a 2 years period [30]. Authors suggested that patients are oftenly referred to late to surgery and that an earlier intervention may improve immediate and possibly midterm outcomes. Nevertheless, this hypothesis has not been proved yet. As a result, in the real-world setting, TV surgery for isolated TR is rarely performed and therefore, most patients are managed conservatively.

3. Transcatheter therapies for tricuspid regurgitation

Given the unmet need for invasive correction of TR with an assumable procedural risk, different percutaneous devices have been developed in recent years based on previous surgical techniques and percutaneous devices dedicated for the treatment of left-side valve disease. **Table 3** summarizes anatomical target and surgical background, if any, of current available devices for transcatheter treatment of TR, including percutaneous TV repair (PTVR) techniques and orthotopic and heterotopic transcatheter TV valve implantation (TTVI). To date, only 3 devices have already obtain the CE mark for clinical practice [12, 31].

3.1 Percutaneous tricuspid valve repair

3.1.1 Percutaneous coaptation devices

These devices are designed to ultimately minimize the coaptation gap, including: 1) MITRACLIP in the tricuspid position or TRICLIP that approximate the leaflets

	Anatomical target	*Surgical background*	*CE mark*
MITRACLIP/TRICLIP	Leaflets	Edge-to-edge Clover suture	Yes
PASCAL			Yes
FORMA		No	No
MISTRAL	Leaflets + tendinous cords	No	No
CARDIOBAND	Tricuspid valve annulus	Annuloplasty ring	Yes
IRIS MILLIPEDE			No
DA VIGNI			No
TRIALIGN		Kay bicuspidization suture	No
TRICINCH			No
PASTA		Hetzer double orifice suture	No
MIA		Suture annuloplasty	No
TRAIPTA		No	No
NAVIGATE	Tricuspid valve	TVR	No
LUX-VALVE		TVR	No
TRISOL VALVE		TVR	No
SAPIEN	Vena cava	No	No
TRICVALVE		No	No
TRICENTO		No	No

Table 3.
Transcatheter therapies for tricuspid regurgitation.

increasing its coaptation surface; 2) FORMA device, comprising a spacer that occupies the regurgitant orifice; 3) PASCAL, that combines clipping of leaflets with a minor spacer; and 4) the MISTRAL device that approaches leaflets' coaptation edge by stretching the subvalvular apparatus (**Figure 1**).

a. MITRACLIP/TRICLIP

MitraClip (Abbott Vascular, Santa Clara, CA, USA) is a polyester-coated chromium-cobalt device with two arms that open and close in a controlled manner through the release system. The device can be repositioned and more devices can be implanted until an adequate reduction of the valve insufficiency is achieved. This device was initially designed for the percutaneous treatment of mitral regurgitation and has already been used in over 100.000 for this purpose. With this back up of experience gained in the treatment of mitral regurgitation, it began to be used as an off-label therapy for TR and become the most widely used PTVR device (70% of all procedures).

The TriValve registry evaluated the results of MitraClip at 1-year follow-up in a series of 249 patients with TR [32]. Concomitant treatment of the mitral valve was carried out in 52% of the cases and two or more clips were implanted in 69.1% of the patients received, most of them (65%) at the anteroseptal commissure (65%). Procedural success, defined as TR reduction to grade ≤ 2+, was achieved in 77% of cases and an improvement in functional class to NYHA ≤ II

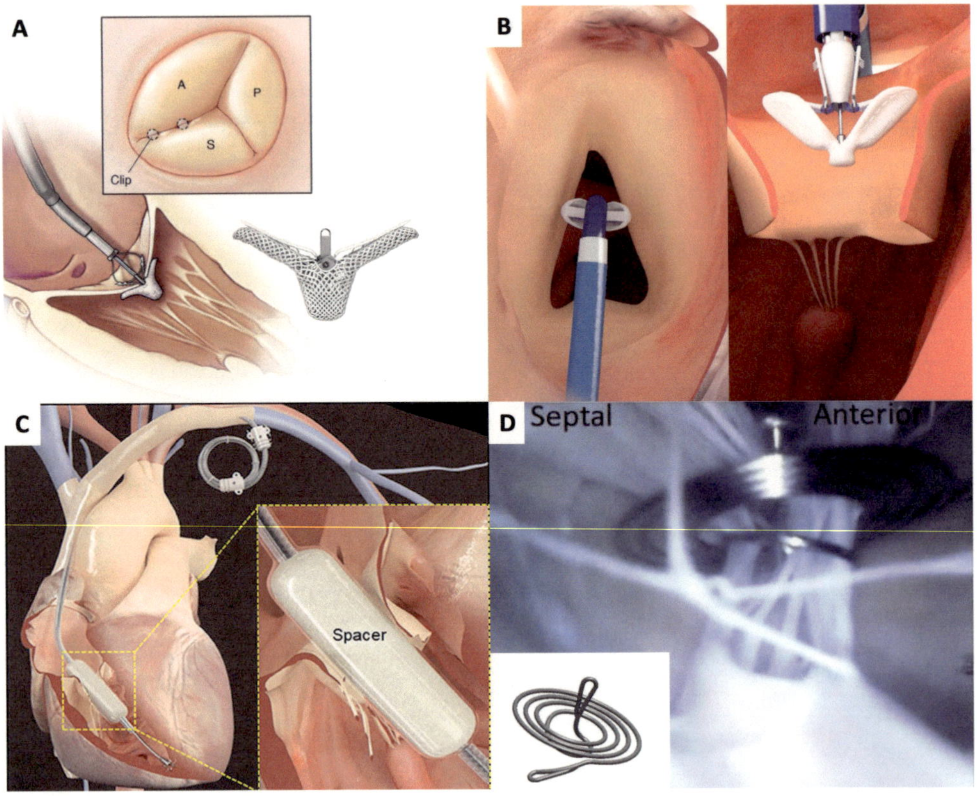

Figure 1.
Tricuspid coaptation devices. A: TRICLIP, B: PASCAL, C: FORMA, D: MISTRAL.

was observed in 69% of patients. The following factors were identified as independent predictors for procedural failure: tenting area > 3.15 cm^2, non-central jet, regurgitation through the anteroposterior or posteroseptal commissure, coaptation gap >6.5 mm and regurgitant area > 0.695 cm^2.

From a technical point of view, two approaches have been described for reducing TR with MitraClip: the triple-orifice technique in which the clips are positioned centrally between the septal and the anterior leaflets, as well as between the septal and the posterior leaflets; and the bicuspidization procedure in which clips are deployed between the anterior and the septal leaflets [33] (**Figure 2**). Clipping of the anteroposterior commissure can be challenging and, sometimes, this may distort the valve and worsen TR [34].

The TriClip (Abbott Vascular, Santa Clara, CA, USA) is a dedicated MitraClip device for the TV. The prospective single-arm multicenter TRILUMINATE study evaluated the safety and feasibility of this system for treating TR. The 6-month results involving 85 patients have recently been published [35]. Patients with severe PH or relevant mitral valve insufficiency were excluded. Technical success was achieved in all the patients and most clips were deployed between the anterior and septal leaflets (77%) with a reduction of at least one grade in the severity of TR in 91% of the cases. At 6-month follow-up, 86% of the patients presented moderate or less TR and were in NYHA functional class was I-II, and a significant improvement in the 6-minute walking test was observed.

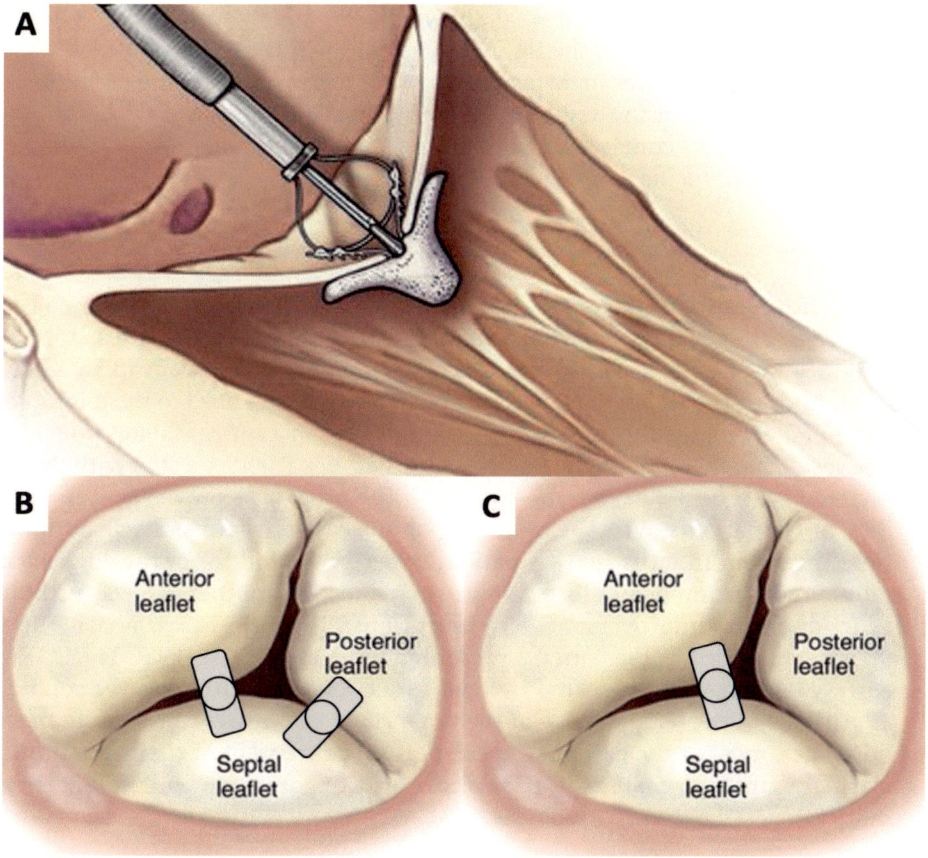

Figure 2.
A: Percutaneous tricuspid valve repair with MitraClip. B: Triple-orifice technique. C: Bicuspidization aproach.

Patients with significant TR and implantable cardiac devices represent a particularly challenging population. In a cohort of the TriValve registry, PTVR was performed in 121 patients with an intracardiac RV electrodes. Most of these patients, 106 (87%), were treated with MitraClip and compare to those without intracardiac devices, no significant differences were documented in procedural success, TR reduction (TR ≤ 2+ 73.7% vs. 70.8%, p = 0.6), clinical improvement or survival [36].

b. PASCAL

The Pascal system combines the possibility of grasping the leaflets as with the MitraClip device with the use of a spacer. This affords improved coaptation and better outcomes following percutaneous repair of TR. The first experience targeted to the tricuspid valve in humans have recently been published [37]. Out of 28 patients (98% with functional TR), the procedure success rate was 86%, with no complications in any case. Forty devices were implanted - mostly in the anteroseptal position (70%). Detachment of the device was recorded in two patients, and 85% of the subjects presented TR ≤ 2+ after 30 days.

Although no clinical trials have compared any of these therapies versus placebo in patients with TR, an observational study has compared the use of the MitraClip with the PASCAL system in the treatment of this valve disease. In this study published by Braun et al., in which 88 patients were treated with the MitraClip and 32 received the PASCAL system, no differences were observed between the two devices in terms of success of the procedure, the reduction of TR or detachment of the device (11% with MitraClip versus 6% with PASCAL). The authors concluded that both devices are similar in terms of efficacy and safety in reducing TR [38].

c. FORMA

The FORMA system (Edwards Lifesciences, Irvine, CA, USA) is designed to increase leaflet coaptation, occupying the regurgitant orifice with a spacer [39]. A guide is advanced through the subclavian or axillary vein and anchored in the apex of the right ventricle. The spacer is then advanced to the tricuspid valve plane. Finally, the excess guide is implanted in a subcutaneous pouch. The results after 2–3 years of the first cohort of 19 patients treated with this system have recently been published [40]. The procedure proved successful in 89% of the patients, with the recording of one case of right ventricle perforation. After four months another patient suffered thrombosis of the device, and pulmonary thromboembolism was also evidenced in another subject. Although functional class improvement was observed in 93% of the cases, at last follow-up only one-third of the patients presented moderate or lesser TR. The FORMA early feasibility study reported two right ventricle perforations in the cohort of 29 patients. A decrease in TR was seen in 49% of the cases [40]. Despite these outcomes, most of the patients experienced improvement of their functional class. The single-arm SPACER trial is currently ongoing and will evaluate mortality after 30 days with this device.

d. MISTRAL

The results of the first experience in humans with the Mistral device (Mitralix, Yokneam, Israel) have recently been published [41]. This device consists of a spiral nitinol guide that grasps the tendinous cords, approximating them to the leaflets and thus increasing coaptation. This study included 7 patients with severe functional TR; one of them required two devices. No adverse events related to the procedure were recorded after 30 days, and a significant decrease in effective regurgitant orifice area (EROA), vena contracta and regurgitant volume was achieved, together with improved functional class.

3.1.2 Percutaneous annuloplasty devices

As it has been explained above, the basic mechanism underlying functional TR is TVA dilatation, which mainly occurs in its anteroseptal diameter. TV annuloplasty is currently the surgical treatment of choice in this scenario. Based on this surgical technique, different percutaneous annuloplasty devices have been developed in recent years with the fundamental aim of reducing the annular dimensions and prevent further TVA dilatation. These devices can be classified into rings (CARDIOBAND, IRIS MILLIPEDE, DA VIGNI, TRAIPTA) or direct suture devices (TRIALIGN, TRICINCH, PASTA, MIA) (**Figure 3**).

a. CARDIOBAND

The CARDIOBAND (Edwards Lifesciences, Irvine, CA, USA) is an annuloplasty system consisting of an adjustable surgical-like Dacron ring that is im-

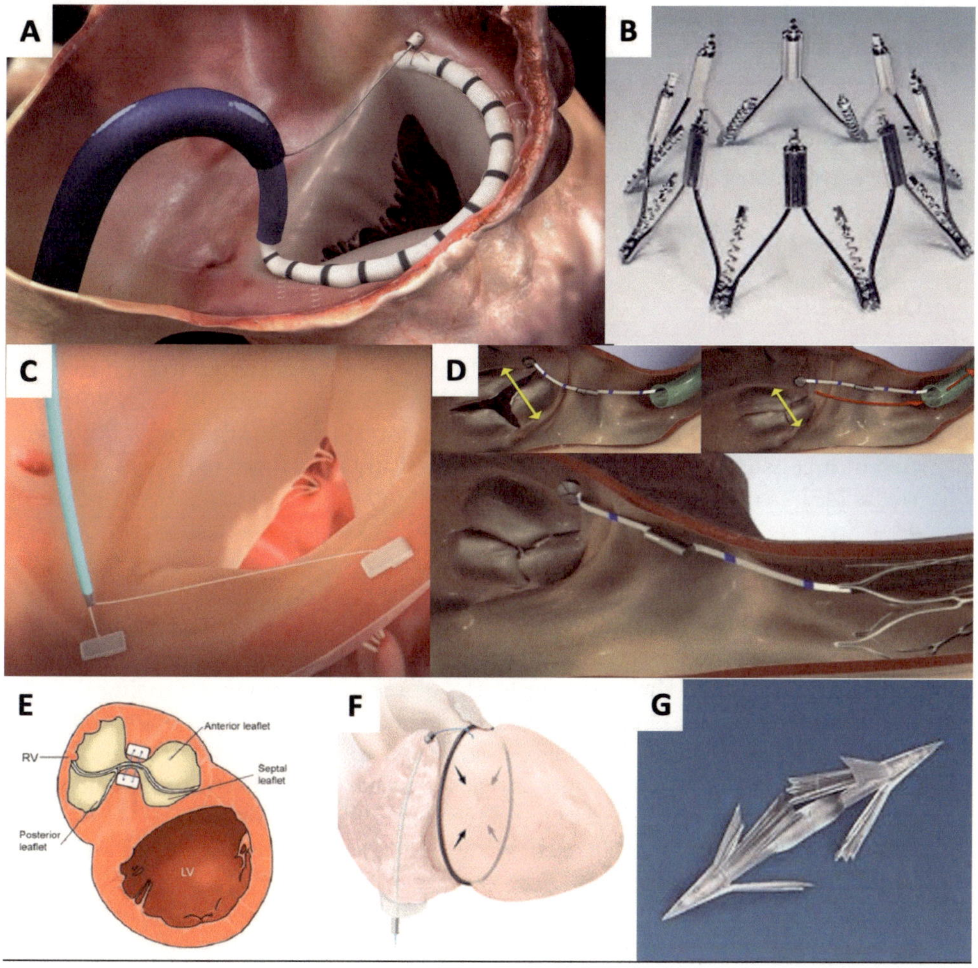

Figure 3.
A: CARDIOBAND, B: Iris MILLIPEDE, C: TRIALIGN, D: TRICINCH, E: Pasta, F: TRAIPTA, G: Mia.

planted on the atrial side of the tricuspid TVA and fixed with multiple anchors. Once the last anchoring has been placed, the device is cinched until enough TR reduction is achieved. The two-year results of the TRI-REPAIR study have recently been published. This trial evaluated the efficacy and safety of this system in 30 patients with symptomatic functional TR (83% in NYHA functional class III-IV) [42]. The procedure was successful in all patients and related to a significant reduction in TR (72% of the subjects presented TR ≤ moderate) and TVA dimension, and to an improvement in functional status (82% of the subjects were in NYHA class I-II), 6-minute walk distance and quality of life at 24-months follow-up. The Early Feasibility Study of CARDIOBAND included 22 patients with severe symptomatic TR in which this treatment was carried out [43]. The procedure success rate was 96%, with improvement of both the severity of TR and of the NYHA functional class.

b. IRIS MILLIPEDE

The IRIS transcatheter annuloplasty system (Boston Scientific, Marlborough, MA), is a complete semirigid ring that is placed in a supra-annular position and anchored through 7–9 screws. The ring can be adjusted to reduce the

TVA diameter and thus the severity of TR. Although this system was initially designed to be used in the mitral valve, Rogers et al. presented the results obtained in two patients that received this device in the tricuspid position in a combined procedure with the mitral valve annuloplasty [44]. For the TV treatment, only 7 of the 9 anchors were used in order to avoid the risk of atrioventricular block. The results in these patients were good showed no need for a pacemaker and a 40% reduction of the TVA size after 12 months, with no residual significant TR.

c. DA VINGI

The DA VINGI is a percutaneous annuloplasty device designed to treat the mitral and tricuspid valves. This device allows complete annuloplasty with a single-step implant. Following a healing period (90 days), the ring is adjusted percutaneously. The device has been successfully implanted to date in 6 patients [45].

d. TRIALING

The TRIALING (Mitralign Inc., Tewksbury, MA, USA) is a direct suture device that reproduces the Kay tricuspid bicuspidization surgical technique leading to the obliteration of the posterior leaflet of the TV. Through a transjugular percutaneous access, two pledgets are inserted in the anteroposterior and posteroseptal commissures. The pledgets are then approximated with a cinching mechanism, bringing both commissures together and obliterating the posterior leaflet. The first published experience corresponds to 14 patients with moderate to severe functional TR, achieving a 51% decrease in EROA and a 34% reduction of the TVA area [46]. The early feasibility SCOUT I trial included 15 patients with functional TR and the device was successfully implanted in all patients [47]. One patient required right coronary angioplasty due to extrinsic compression. At 30-days follow-up, 3 single-pledget annular detachment were documented without reintervention. In the remaining 12 cases, a significant reduction in the TVA area and EROA were observed, together with clinical improvement in functional status [47]. After 12 months, only one patient required surgery. The SCOUT II study is currently ongoing and will include 60 patients [48].

e. TRICINCH

The TriCinch (4Tech Cardio, Galway, Ireland) is an annuloplasty system that consists of a screw for anchoring to the TVA at its supravalvular anterior area and a Dacron band attached to an expandable stent that is placed at the inferior vena cava (IVC), generating tension and thus reducing the diameter of the septolateral diameter of the TVA. In the PREVENT study, 24 patients were treated with the first generation of this device. Implantation success was achieved in 81% of the patients, with a reduction of one grade or more in the severity of TR in 94% of the cases, together with functional class improvement. However, two patients suffered hemopericardium and 5 late detachments were recorded. Because of this, the second-generation TriCinch was developed, incorporating an improved anchoring coil system that is inserted in the pericardial space with two hemostatic seals. The first in-human experience suggests that the device is safe.

f. PASTA

Lastly, the Pledget-assisted suture tricuspid annuloplasty (PASTA) device is an annuloplasty system that reproduces Hetzer's double orifice suture technique. Two sutures are placed at ring level in its anterolateral and posteroseptal portion, with tightening and approximation of the extremities, creating a tricuspid valve with two orifices similar to the final outcome obtained after percutaneous mitral valve repair with the MitraClip device. The first experience was obtained in a porcine model, with good results [49]. The first experience in humans has recently been published, evidencing a marked reduction in valve area - though dehiscence of the device occurred after two days, with the recurrence of TR [50].

g. MIA

The Minimally Invasive Annuloplasty (MIA, Micro Interventional Devices, Newtown, PA, USA) system is a sutureless device with two anchorages that allow reduction of the tricuspid ring. The STTAR study will include 40 patients and will evaluate the efficacy and safety of this device [51].

h. TRAIPTA

The transatrial intrapericardial tricuspid annuloplasty (TRAIPTA) system is an external indirect annuloplasty device. It consists of an adjustable nitinol guide that is advanced through the inferior vena cava to the atrium and penetrating the pericardium through a puncture in the right appendage. Once within the pericardial space, it is positioned in the atrioventricular sulcus, adjusting its size and thus reducing the diameter of the tricuspid ring and improving coaptation of the leaflets. The first experience was with a porcine model, in which a decrease in TR was achieved, with improvement of coaptation and reduction of the diameter of the ring, without serious complications [52]. The puncture zone was sealed with an atrial septal occluder (Amplatzer, St. Jude Medical, St. Paul, Minnesota or Lepu Medical, Beijing, China) in all cases. Although no results in humans are yet available, a new version of the device will be evaluated in a feasibility trial in the coming years.

3.2 Percutaneous tricuspid valve replacement

3.2.1 Orthotopic tricuspid valve implantation

Orthotopic TTVI implies TV replacement and the prosthesis is anchored to the native ring and leaflets. To date, there are three devices available: GATE, LUX-VALVE, TRISOL and EVOQUE (**Figure 4A-C**).

a. GATE

The GATE (NaviGate Cardiac Structures, Lake Forest, CA, USA) is a self-expanding valve dedicated for placement in the tricuspid position. This is a conical shaped device with three pericardial leaflets surrounded by a nitinol stent that has twelve atrial winglets and ventricular graspers to ensure anchoring. The device comes in 5 different sizes (36, 40, 44, 48 and 52 mm in diameter) and the procedure can be performed via transjugular or through a minithoracot-

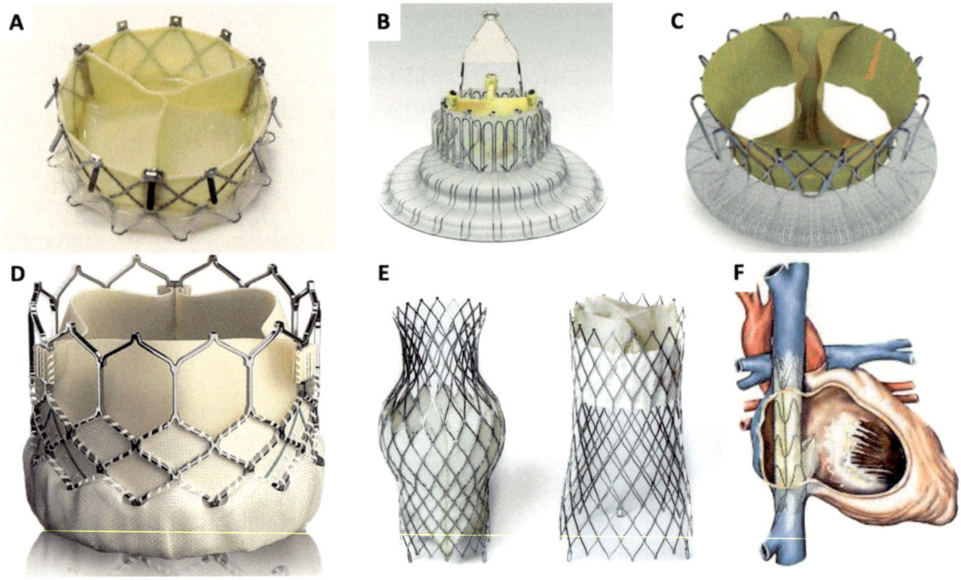

Figure 4.
A: Gate, B: Lux-valve, C: TRISOL, D: Edwards SAPIEN, E: TRICVALVE, F: TRICENTO.

omy access. The first reported compassionate use of this system in 35 patients recorded a procedural success rate of 76%, with residual TR ≤ 2+ in all cases, and need for surgery in 14% with a 14% 30-day mortality [53]. A multicenter registry has been recently published including 30 patients with severe TR and right ventricular dysfunction in which the GATE system [54]. Technical success was achieved in 87%, but device malpositioning occurred in 4 patients, with conversion to open heart surgery in 2 of them (5%). Among those who received the device, 76% had mild or less TR at discharge with an in-hospital mortality was 10%. In addition, at 6-months follow-up, 62% of the patients were in NYHA I or II with no late device-related adverse events were documented.

b. LUX-VALVE

LUX-Valve (Jenscare Biotechnology, Ningbo, China) is a self-expanding valve that is inserted through the right atrium via a minithoracotomy and anchored throught a dedicated mechanism to the leaflets and the interventricular septum. Lu et al. published their first-in-human experience in 12 patients with severe TR and functional class IV [55]. The procedure was successful in all patients, but one patient required surgery due to bleeding and another died of an acute myocardial infarction. A decrease in TR was observed in all cases, with only one of them with a residual moderate leak. The largest series to date with results from 35 patients with severe TR and functional class III/IV has recently been communicated [56]. The mortality rate at 30 days was 5.7%, with significant clinical improvement in NYHA functional class and a decrease in right ventricle volume.

c. TRISOL

The TriSol (TriSol Medical, Yokneam, Israel) is a valve specifically designed for the treatment of TR that is still in the preclinical development phase.

d. EVOQUE

The EVOQUE valve (Edwards Lifesciences, Irvine, CA) was recently evaluated in 25 symptomatic (96% NYHA III or IV) patients with severe TR. At 30 days 76% of the patients were in NYHA I/II and 96% had a TR 2+ with a 92% of technical success [57].

3.2.2 Heterotopic tricuspid valve implantation

Heterotopic TTVI refers to the implantation of a competent valve in a position different from the native tricuspid valve. The inferior vena cava (IVC), generally in combination with the superior vena cava (SVC), are the sites of choice, leading to the ventricularization of the right atrium [17]. Therefore, this approach does not address the TR itself, but prevents from severe systemic venous congestion related to right HF. As a palliative therapy, is it usually indicated in severely symptomatic patients with end-stage HF and massive or torrential TR not deemed candidates for other invasive approaches. Compared with orthotopic TTVI, this procedure is simpler, avoids the introduction of prosthetic material in the inlet of the RV and the position of the valve does not interfere with pacemaker or defibrillator electrodes, if present [58]. On the contrary, clinical impact of untreated TR, right atrial ventricularization, persistent right atrial volume overload and potentially increased RV afterload is unknown. This group of devices includes SAPIEN, TRICVALVE and TRICENTO (**Figure 4D–F**).

a. SAPIEN

The SAPIEN (Edwards Lifesciences, Irvine, CA, USA) is a triple-leaflet bovine pericardium valve initially designed for aortic valve replacement in patients with severe aortic stenosis. The first off-label use of the SAPIEN XT in the IVC was published in 2013 in three patients [59]. After that initial experience, this technique was tested in a randomized controlled trial that included 28 patients comparing medical treatment versus percutaneous implantation of this valve in the IVC. The main endpoint of the trial was the exercise capacity evaluated by cardiopulmonary exercise test. Nevertheless, this study had to be suspended prematurely due to futility and to the recording of numerous complications in the device group [60]. The analysis of available data evidenced a systolic decrease in the hepatic vein flow, without reverse RV remodeling [61]. In a recent retrospective multicenter registry enrolling 25 patients with severe symptomatic TR undergoing heterotopic TTVI (72% SAPIEN XT/3, 24% TRICVALVE and 4% DIRECTFLOW) in the IVC (76%) or both VC (24%), the procedure was successful in 96% of the patients although in-hospital mortality was 16% [62].

b. TRICVALVE

The TRICVALVE (P&F Products & Features, Vienna, Austria) is a device specifically designed for its implantation in VC. It consists of two self-expanding bovine pericardium valves on a nitinol stent, one for each VC. Lauten et al. published first in-human experience in 2011 in a patient that showed clinical functional improvement after 8 weeks [63]. The TRICUS feasibility study is currently ongoing and will include 10 patients in order to evaluate of clinical and adverse events using this device [NCT03723239].

c. TRICENTO

The Tricento (NVT, Muri, Switzerland) is a coated bicaval covered stent with a bicuspid valve positioned laterally that that allows inflow into the right atrium. Since the first experience reported in 2018 [64], isolated cases have been published, with good periprocedural results [65, 66].

3.3 Outcomes after transcatheter tricuspid valve therapies

3.3.1 Clinical benefits

Most feasibility studies and observational registries have shown a significant clinical improvement in terms of NYHA functional class, quality of life or 6-minute walk test in patients undergoing PTVR or TTVI. These changes were observed even after conservative reductions of TR of 1 or 2 grades after PTVR. Nevertheless, no data are available from randomized controlled trials comparing percutaneous approach with medical management, and current reported follow-up does not exceed 1 or 2 years after the invasive procedure.

With regard to cardiovascular events, Orban et al. evaluated rates of admissions due to HF in 119 patients undergoing isolated PTVR (MitraClip 97%) comparing the year before and after the procedure [67]. PTVR was associated with a significant reduction in the grade of TR to moderate or less in 72% of the cases and with a significant lesser incidence of HF admissions ($p = 0.02$).

Recently, results from the TriValve registry that included 312 patients mostly treated with MitraClip device, reported that 30-day mortality was significantly lower among those with procedural success (1.9% vs. 6.9%, $p = 0.04$) [68]. Furthermore, more recently, Taramasso et al. published a retrospective propensity matched case–control study that included 268 patients from the same registry who underwent PTVR and observed significant lower 1-year mortality (23 ± 3% vs. 36 ± 3%, $p = 0.001$) and rehospitalization (26 ± 3% vs. 47 ± 3%, $p < 0.0001$) rates when compared to controls managed conservatively [69]. In addition, those patients treated with PTVR had higher survival after adjusted for sex, NYHA functional class, right ventricular dysfunction and AF. Although these results are encouraging, potential survival benefit of transcatheter tricuspid valve interventions over stand-alone medical therapy needs to be tested in clinical trials. Currently, diverse ongoing randomized trials will assess this issue in patients receiving TriClip, Pascal, Cardioband, and other PTVR devices.

3.3.2 Predictors of outcomes

One of the major limitations of TV surgery is reported high periprocedural mortality. Despite transcatheter approaches seem to significantly reduce this risk, patient selection remains key to achieve optimal procedural and clinical results. In this regard, some important determinants of outcomes have ben already suggested:

a. PH and RV function: Lurz et al. evaluated invasive pulmonary artery pressures and echocardiographic parameters in 243 patients who underwent PTVR [70]. The presence of invasive PH, defined as pulmonary artery systolic pressure > 50 mmHg), together with discordant absence of PH by echocardiographic estimation, was associated with the combined primary endpoint of all-cause mortality, need for repeat hospitalization for HF and reintervention during follow-up. This could be explained because in advanced stages of TR associated with adverse RV remodeling with severe dilation of the TV annulus, pulmonary hypertension may be severely underestimated by echocardiography. Moreover, Stocker et al. observed in a multicenter study including 236 patients that invasive mean pulmonary artery pressure, transpulmonary gradient, pulmonary vascular resistance and RV stroke work were significant predictors of 1-year mortality, and that patients with pre-capillary PH had the worse prognosis [71]. Similarly, the ratio between TAPSE/invasive PH <0.29 mm/mmHg has also shown adverse prognosis impact [72]. This finding points out the close relationship between the RV function and PH. So-called RV-PA coupling refers to the fact that RV contractility should "match" the RV afterload.

b. Nutritional status: from a clinical perspective, a recent study reported that an impaired nutritional status is also associated with an increased risk of death and rehospitalization for heart failure after PTVR [73]. This finding is important since to date most patients were referred to invasive management at an advance stage of RV failure in which nutritional status might be already impaired and this can impact outcomes.

3.3.3 Patient and device selection

The decision-making process for patient and device selection in these early stages of percutaneous approaches to treat TR prompts exhaustive clinical evaluation, specifically guided right heart catheterization and transesophageal hemodynamic and anatomical evaluation, and heart team meeting. **Figure 5** summarizes a theorical approach.

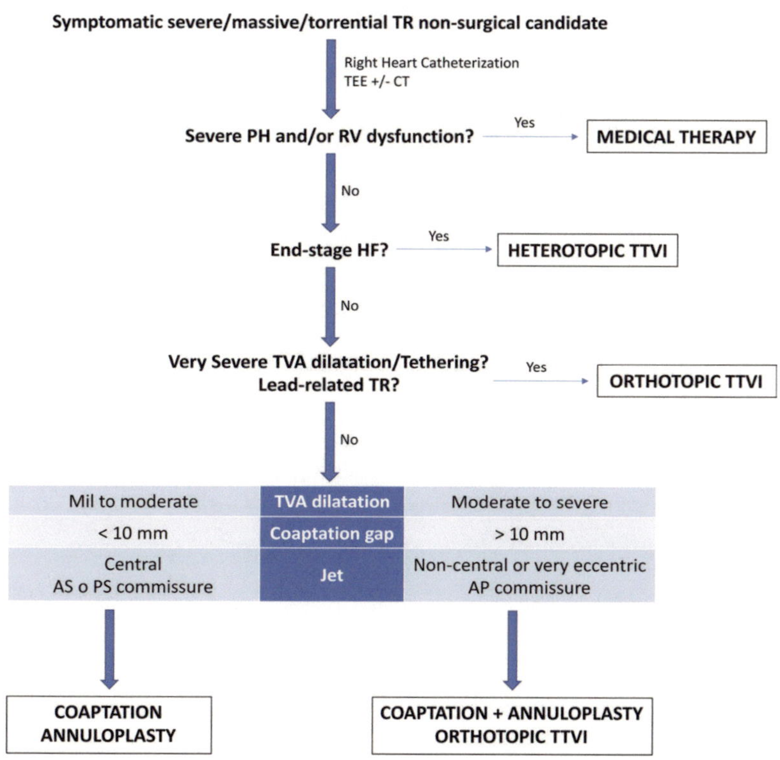

Figure 5.
Theorical algorithm for device selection. TTVI: Transcatheter tricuspid valve implantation, AP: Anteroseptal, PS: Posteroseptal, AP: Anteroposterior.

4. Conclusions

TR is a common heart valve disease associated with high morbidity and mortality when conservatively managed. Surgery is currently the treatment of choice, though very few patients with isolated TR undergo TV surgery in the real-world setting due to high surgical risk. In recent years, different percutaneous treatment devices have been developed offering promising results with much lower procedural adverse outcomes. Further studies are needed to find which will benefit the most from these therapies.

Conflict of interest

Rodrigo Estévez and Carmen Garrote are proctors for MitraClip.

Appendices and Nomenclature

AF	Atrial Fibrillation
CHD	Congenital Heart Disease
EMB	Endomyocardial biopsy
EROA	Effective Regurgitant Orifice Area
FAC	Fractional Area Change
ICD	Implantable Cardiac Device
MIA	Minimally Invasive Annuloplasty
PAP	Pulmonary Artery Pressure
PASTA	Pledget-assisted suture tricuspid annuloplasty
PH	Pulmonary hypertension
PTVR	Percutaneous Tricuspid Valve Repair
RV	Right ventricle
TAPSE	Tricuspid Annular Plane Systolic Excursion
TR	Tricuspid Regurgitation
TRAIPTA	Transatrial Intrapericardial Tricuspid Annuloplasty
TTVI	Transcatheter Tricuspid Valve Implantation
TV	Tricuspid valve
TVA	Tricuspid Valve Annulus
VC	vena contracta
3D VCA	three-dimensional vena contracta área

Author details

Carlos Minguito-Carazo[1], Tomás Benito-González[1*], Rodrigo Estévez-Loureiro[2], Carmen Garrote-Coloma[1], Julio Echarte-Morales[1], Armando Pérez de Prado[1] and Felipe Fernández-Vázquez[1]

1 Department of Cardiology, University Hospital of León, León, Spain

2 Department of Cardiology, University Hospital Alvaro Cunqueiro, Vigo, Spain

*Address all correspondence to: tomasbenito@outlook.com

References

[1] Demir OM, Regazzoli D, Mangieri A, Ancona MB, Mitomo S, Weisz G, et al. Transcatheter Tricuspid Valve Replacement: Principles and Design [Internet]. Vol. 5, Frontiers in Cardiovascular Medicine. Frontiers Media S.A.; 2018 [cited 2020 Dec 10]. Available from: https://pubmed.ncbi.nlm.nih.gov/30283790/

[2] Singh JP, Evans JC, Levy D, Larson MG, Freed LA, Fuller DL, et al. Prevalence and clinical determinants of mitral, tricuspid, and aortic regurgitation (The Framingham Heart Study). Am J Cardiol [Internet]. 1999 Mar 15 [cited 2020 Dec 10];83(6):897-902. Available from: https://pubmed.ncbi.nlm.nih.gov/10190406/

[3] Rodés-Cabau J, Taramasso M, O'Gara PT. Diagnosis and treatment of tricuspid valve disease: current and future perspectives [Internet]. Vol. 388, The Lancet. Lancet Publishing Group; 2016 [cited 2020 Dec 10]. p. 2431-42. Available from: https://pubmed.ncbi.nlm.nih.gov/27048553/

[4] Wang N, Fulcher J, Abeysuriya N, McGrady M, Wilcox I, Celermajer D, et al. Tricuspid regurgitation is associated with increased mortality independent of pulmonary pressures and right heart failure: A systematic review and meta-analysis. Eur Heart J [Internet]. 2019 [cited 2020 Dec 10];40(5):476-84. Available from: https://pubmed.ncbi.nlm.nih.gov/30351406/

[5] Topilsky Y, Nkomo VT, Vatury O, Michelena HI, Letourneau T, Suri RM, et al. Clinical outcome of isolated tricuspid regurgitation. JACC Cardiovasc Imaging [Internet]. 2014 [cited 2020 Dec 10];7(12):1185-94. Available from: https://pubmed.ncbi.nlm.nih.gov/25440592/

[6] Stuge O, Liddicoat J. Emerging opportunities for cardiac surgeons within structural heart disease [Internet]. Vol. 132, Journal of Thoracic and Cardiovascular Surgery. J Thorac Cardiovasc Surg; 2006 [cited 2020 Dec 10]. p. 1258-61. Available from: https://pubmed.ncbi.nlm.nih.gov/17140937/

[7] Zack CJ, Fender EA, Chandrashekar P, Reddy YNV, Bennett CE, Stulak JM, et al. National Trends and Outcomes in Isolated Tricuspid Valve Surgery. J Am Coll Cardiol [Internet]. 2017 Dec 19 [cited 2020 Dec 10];70(24):2953-60. Available from: https://pubmed.ncbi.nlm.nih.gov/29241483/

[8] Alqahtani F, Berzingi CO, Aljohani S, Hijazi M, Al-Hallak A, Alkhouli M. Contemporary Trends in the Use and Outcomes of Surgical Treatment of Tricuspid Regurgitation. J Am Heart Assoc [Internet]. 2017 Dec 22 [cited 2020 Dec 10];6(12). Available from: https://pubmed.ncbi.nlm.nih.gov/29273638/

[9] Kawada N, Naganuma H, Muramatsu K, Ishibashi-Ueda H, Bando K, Hashimoto K. Redefinition of tricuspid valve structures for successful ring annuloplasty. J Thorac Cardiovasc Surg [Internet]. 2018 Apr 1 [cited 2020 Dec 10];155(4):1511-1519.e1. Available from: https://pubmed.ncbi.nlm.nih.gov/29366576/

[10] Athavale S, Deopujari R, Sinha U, Lalwani R, Kotgirwar S. Is tricuspid valve really tricuspid? Anat Cell Biol [Internet]. 2017 Mar 1 [cited 2020 Dec 10];50(1):1-6. Available from: https://pubmed.ncbi.nlm.nih.gov/28417048/

[11] Lama P, Tamang BK, Kulkarni J. Morphometry and aberrant morphology of the adult human tricuspid valve leaflets. Anat Sci Int [Internet]. 2016 Mar 1 [cited 2020 Dec 10];91(2):143-50. Available from: https://pubmed.ncbi.nlm.nih.gov/25677415/

[12] Santaló-Corcoy M, Asmarats L, Li C-H, Arzamendi D. Catheter-based treatment of tricuspid regurgitation: state of the art. Ann Transl Med [Internet]. 2020 Aug [cited 2020 Dec 10];8(15):964-964. Available from: https://pubmed.ncbi.nlm.nih.gov/32953764/

[13] Taramasso M, Maisano F. Novel Technologies for percutaneous treatment of tricuspid valve regurgitation. Eur Heart J [Internet]. 2017 Sep 21 [cited 2020 Dec 10];38(36):2707-10. Available from: https://pubmed.ncbi.nlm.nih.gov/29044389/

[14] Chang CC, Veen KM, Hahn RT, Bogers AJJC, Latib A, Oei FBS, et al. Uncertainties and challenges in surgical and transcatheter tricuspid valve therapy: A state-of-the-art expert review [Internet]. Vol. 41, European Heart Journal. Oxford University Press; 2020 [cited 2020 Dec 10]. p. 1932-40. Available from: https://pubmed.ncbi.nlm.nih.gov/31511897/

[15] Rogers JH, Bolling SF. The tricuspid valve: Current perspective and evolving management of tricuspid regurgitation. Circulation [Internet]. 2009 May 26 [cited 2017 Jan 29];119(20):2718-25. Available from: http://www.ncbi.nlm.nih.gov/pubmed/19470900

[16] Badano LP, Muraru D, Enriquez-Sarano M. Assessment of functional tricuspid regurgitation [Internet]. Vol. 34, European Heart Journal. Eur Heart J; 2013 [cited 2020 Dec 10]. p. 1875-84. Available from: https://pubmed.ncbi.nlm.nih.gov/23303656/

[17] Mangieri A, Montalto C, Pagnesi M, Jabbour RJ, Rodés-Cabau J, Moat N, et al. Mechanism and Implications of the Tricuspid Regurgitation: From the Pathophysiology to the Current and Future Therapeutic Options [Internet]. Vol. 10, Circulation: Cardiovascular Interventions. Lippincott Williams and Wilkins; 2017 [cited 2020 Dec 10]. Available from: https://pubmed.ncbi.nlm.nih.gov/28698289/

[18] Utsunomiya H, Itabashi Y, Mihara H, Berdejo J, Kobayashi S, Siegel RJ, et al. Functional Tricuspid Regurgitation Caused by Chronic Atrial Fibrillation: A Real-Time 3-Dimensional Transesophageal Echocardiography Study. Circ Cardiovasc Imaging [Internet]. 2017 Jan 1 [cited 2020 Dec 10];10(1). Available from: https://pubmed.ncbi.nlm.nih.gov/28073806/

[19] Taramasso M, Calen C, Guidotti A, Kuwata S, Biefer HRC, Nietlispach F, et al. Management of tricuspid regurgitation: The role of transcatheter therapies. Interv Cardiol Rev [Internet]. 2017 Mar 1 [cited 2020 Dec 10];12(1):51-5. Available from: /pmc/articles/PMC5808466/?report=abstract

[20] Zoghbi WA, Adams D, Bonow RO, Enriquez-Sarano M, Foster E, Grayburn PA, et al. Recommendations for Noninvasive Evaluation of Native Valvular Regurgitation: A Report from the American Society of Echocardiography Developed in Collaboration with the Society for Cardiovascular Magnetic Resonance. J Am Soc Echocardiogr [Internet]. 2017 Apr [cited 2018 Mar 11];30(4):303-71. Available from: http://www.ncbi.nlm.nih.gov/pubmed/28314623

[21] Hahn RT, Zamorano JL. The need for a new tricuspid regurgitation grading scheme [Internet]. Vol. 18, European Heart Journal Cardiovascular Imaging. Oxford University Press; 2017 [cited 2020 Dec 10]. p. 1342-3. Available from: https://pubmed.ncbi.nlm.nih.gov/28977455/

[22] Santoro C, Marco Del Castillo A, González-Gómez A, Monteagudo JM, Hinojar R, Lorente A, et al. Mid-term outcome of severe tricuspid

regurgitation: Are there any differences according to mechanism and severity? Eur Heart J Cardiovasc Imaging [Internet]. 2019 Sep 1 [cited 2020 Dec 10];20(9):1035-42. Available from: https://pubmed.ncbi.nlm.nih.gov/30830219/

[23] Prihadi EA, Van Der Bijl P, Dietz M, Abou R, Vollema EM, Marsan NA, et al. Prognostic Implications of Right Ventricular Free Wall Longitudinal Strain in Patients With Significant Functional Tricuspid Regurgitation. Circ Cardiovasc Imaging [Internet]. 2019 Mar 1 [cited 2020 Dec 10];12(3). Available from: https://pubmed.ncbi.nlm.nih.gov/30879327/

[24] Khalique OK, Cavalcante JL, Shah D, Guta AC, Zhan Y, Piazza N, et al. Multimodality Imaging of the Tricuspid Valve and Right Heart Anatomy [Internet]. Vol. 12, JACC: Cardiovascular Imaging. Elsevier Inc.; 2019 [cited 2020 Dec 10]. p. 516-31. Available from: https://pubmed.ncbi.nlm.nih.gov/30846125/

[25] Nath J, Foster E, Heidenreich PA. Impact of Tricuspid Regurgitation on Long-Term Survival. J Am Coll Cardiol [Internet]. 2004 Feb 4 [cited 2020 Dec 10];43(3):405-9. Available from: https://pubmed.ncbi.nlm.nih.gov/15013122/

[26] Chorin E, Rozenbaum Z, Topilsky Y, Konigstein M, Ziv-Baran T, Richert E, et al. Tricuspid regurgitation and long-term clinical outcomes. Eur Heart J Cardiovasc Imaging [Internet]. 2020 Sep 23 [cited 2020 Dec 10];21(2):157-65. Available from: https://academic.oup.com/ehjcimaging/advance-article/doi/10.1093/ehjci/jez216/5572606

[27] Topilsky Y, Nkomo VT, Vatury O, Michelena HI, Letourneau T, Suri RM, et al. Clinical outcome of isolated tricuspid regurgitation. JACC Cardiovasc Imaging [Internet]. 2014 Dec [cited 2017 Jan 29];7(12):1185-94. Available from: http://linkinghub.elsevier.com/retrieve/pii/S1936878X14007372

[28] Wang TKM, Griffin BP, Miyasaka R, Xu B, Popovic ZB, Pettersson GB, et al. Isolated surgical tricuspid repair versus replacement: Meta-analysis of 15 069 patients. Open Hear [Internet]. 2020 Mar 17 [cited 2020 Dec 10];7(1):1227. Available from: http://openheart.bmj.com/

[29] Parolari A, Barili F, Pilozzi A, Pacini D. Ring or suture annuloplasty for tricuspid regurgitation? A meta-analysis review [Internet]. Vol. 98, Annals of Thoracic Surgery. Elsevier USA; 2014 [cited 2020 Dec 10]. p. 2255-63. Available from: https://pubmed.ncbi.nlm.nih.gov/25443026/

[30] Dreyfus GD, Corbi PJ, Chan KMJ, Bahrami T. Secondary tricuspid regurgitation or dilatation: Which should be the criteria for surgical repair? Ann Thorac Surg [Internet]. 2005 Jan [cited 2020 Dec 10];79(1):127-32. Available from: https://pubmed.ncbi.nlm.nih.gov/15620928/

[31] Kolte D, Elmariah S. Current state of transcatheter tricuspid valve repair [Internet]. Vol. 10, Cardiovascular Diagnosis and Therapy. AME Publishing Company; 2020 [cited 2020 Dec 11]. p. 89-97. Available from: https://pubmed.ncbi.nlm.nih.gov/32175231/

[32] Mehr M, Taramasso M, Besler C, Ruf T, Connelly KA, Weber M, et al. 1-Year Outcomes After Edge-to-Edge Valve Repair for Symptomatic Tricuspid Regurgitation: Results From the TriValve Registry. JACC Cardiovasc Interv [Internet]. 2019 Aug 12 [cited 2020 Dec 11];12(15):1451-61. Available from: https://pubmed.ncbi.nlm.nih.gov/31395215/

[33] Braun D, Orban M, Orban M, Hagl C, Massberg S, Nabauer M, et al. Transcatheter Edge-to-Edge Repair

for Severe Tricuspid Regurgitation Using the Triple-Orifice Technique Versus the Bicuspidalization Technique [Internet]. Vol. 11, JACC: Cardiovascular Interventions. Elsevier Inc.; 2018 [cited 2020 Dec 11]. p. 1790-2. Available from: https://pubmed.ncbi.nlm.nih.gov/30170957/

[34] Overtchouk P, Piazza N, Granada J, Soliman O, Prendergast B, Modine T. Advances in transcatheter mitral and tricuspid therapies [Internet]. Vol. 20, BMC Cardiovascular Disorders. BioMed Central Ltd.; 2020 [cited 2020 Dec 11]. p. 1. Available from: https://bmccardiovascdisord.biomedcentral.com/articles/10.1186/s12872-019-01312-3

[35] Nickenig G, Weber M, Lurz P, von Bardeleben RS, Sitges M, Sorajja P, et al. Transcatheter edge-to-edge repair for reduction of tricuspid regurgitation: 6-month outcomes of the TRILUMINATE single-arm study. Lancet [Internet]. 2019 Nov 30 [cited 2020 Dec 10];394(10213):2002-11. Available from: http://www.thelancet.com/article/S0140673619326005/fulltext

[36] Taramasso M, Gavazzoni M, Pozzoli A, Alessandrini H, Latib A, Attinger-Toller A, et al. Outcomes of TTVI in Patients With Pacemaker or Defibrillator Leads: Data From the TriValve Registry. JACC Cardiovasc Interv [Internet]. 2020 Mar 9 [cited 2020 Dec 11];13(5):554-64. Available from: https://pubmed.ncbi.nlm.nih.gov/31954676/

[37] Fam NP, Braun D, von Bardeleben RS, Nabauer M, Ruf T, Connelly KA, et al. Compassionate Use of the PASCAL Transcatheter Valve Repair System for Severe Tricuspid Regurgitation: A Multicenter, Observational, First-in-Human Experience. JACC Cardiovasc Interv [Internet]. 2019 Dec 23 [cited 2020 Dec 11];12(24):2488-95. Available from: https://pubmed.ncbi.nlm.nih.gov/31857018/

[38] Braun D, Löw K, Orban M, Mehr M, Gmeiner J, Massberg S, et al. MITRACLIP XTR VS. PASCAL TRANSCATHETER VALVE REPAIR SYSTEM FOR EDGE-TO-EDGE REPAIR OF SEVERE TRICUSPID REGURGITATION. J Am Coll Cardiol. 2020;

[39] Muntané-Carol G, Alperi A, Faroux L, Bédard E, Philippon F, Rodés-Cabau J. Transcatheter Tricuspid Valve Intervention: Coaptation Devices. Front Cardiovasc Med [Internet]. 2020 Aug 13 [cited 2020 Dec 11];7:139. Available from: https://www.frontiersin.org/article/10.3389/fcvm.2020.00139/full

[40] Asmarats L, Perlman G, Praz F, Hensey M, Chrissoheris MP, Philippon F, et al. Long-Term Outcomes of the FORMA Transcatheter Tricuspid Valve Repair System for the Treatment of Severe Tricuspid Regurgitation: Insights From the First-in-Human Experience. JACC Cardiovasc Interv [Internet]. 2019 Aug 12 [cited 2020 Dec 11];12(15):1438-47. Available from: https://pubmed.ncbi.nlm.nih.gov/31395213/

[41] Planer D, Beeri R, Danenberg HD. First-in-Human Transcatheter Tricuspid Valve Repair: 30-Day Follow-Up Experience With the Mistral Device. JACC Cardiovasc Interv [Internet]. 2020 Sep 28 [cited 2020 Dec 11];13(18):2091-6. Available from: https://pubmed.ncbi.nlm.nih.gov/32972568/

[42] Nickenig G, Weber M, Schüler R, Hausleiter J, Nabauer M, von Bardeleben RS, et al. Two-year Outcomes with the Cardioband Tricuspid System from the Multicentre, Prospective TRI-REPAIR Study. EuroIntervention [Internet]. 2020 Oct 13 [cited 2020 Dec 11]; Available from: https://europepmc.org/article/med/33046437

[43] Davidson C, Lim S, Smith R, Kodali S, Kipperman R, Eleid M, et al. EARLY FEASIBILITY STUDY OF CARDIOBAND TRICUSPID SYSTEM FOR FUNCTIONAL TRICUSPID REGURGITATION: 30 DAY OUTCOMES. J Am Coll Cardiol. 2020;

[44] Rogers JH, Boyd WD, Smith TWR, Ebner AA, Grube E, Bolling SF. Transcatheter Annuloplasty for Mitral Regurgitation with an Adjustable Semi-Rigid Complete Ring: Initial Experience with the Millipede IRIS Device. Struct Hear. 2018;

[45] FiH Study of the DaVingiTM TR System in the Treatment of Patients With Functional Tricuspid Regurgitation.

[46] Yzeiraj E, Sievert H, Nickenig G, Latib A, Hahn R, Schofer J. TCT-86 Early Experience with the Trialign System for Transcatheter Tricuspid Valve Repair: A Multicenter Experience. J Am Coll Cardiol. 2016;

[47] Hahn RT, Meduri CU, Davidson CJ, Lim S, Nazif TM, Ricciardi MJ, et al. Early Feasibility Study of a Transcatheter Tricuspid Valve Annuloplasty: SCOUT Trial 30-Day Results. J Am Coll Cardiol [Internet]. 2017 Apr 11 [cited 2020 Dec 11];69(14):1795-806. Available from: https://pubmed.ncbi.nlm.nih.gov/28385308/

[48] Safety and Performance of the Trialign Percutaneous Tricuspid Valve Annuloplasty System (PTVAS) (SCOUT-II).

[49] Khan JM, Rogers T, Schenke WH, Greenbaum AB, Babaliaros VC, Paone G, et al. Transcatheter pledget-assisted suture tricuspid annuloplasty (PASTA) to create a double-orifice valve. Catheter Cardiovasc Interv [Internet]. 2018 Sep 1 [cited 2020 Dec 11];92(3):E175-84. Available from: https://pubmed.ncbi.nlm.nih.gov/29405564/

[50] Greenbaum AB, Khan JM, Rogers T, Babaliaros VC, Eng MHK, Wang DD, et al. First-in-human transcatheter pledget-assisted suture tricuspid annuloplasty for severe tricuspid insufficiency. Catheter Cardiovasc Interv [Internet]. 2020 [cited 2020 Dec 11]; Available from: https://pubmed.ncbi.nlm.nih.gov/32385950/

[51] Study of Transcatheter Tricuspid Annular Repair (STTAR).

[52] Rogers T, Ratnayaka K, Sonmez M, Franson DN, Schenke WH, Mazal JR, et al. Transatrial intrapericardial tricuspid annuloplasty. JACC Cardiovasc Interv [Internet]. 2015 Mar 1 [cited 2020 Dec 11];8(3):483-91. Available from: https://pubmed.ncbi.nlm.nih.gov/25703872/

[53] Elgharably H, Harb SC, Kapadia S, Svensson LG, Navia JL. Transcatheter innovations in tricuspid regurgitation: Navigate. Progress in Cardiovascular Diseases. 2019.

[54] Hahn RT, Kodali S, Fam N, Bapat V, Bartus K, Rodés-Cabau J, et al. Early Multinational Experience of Transcatheter Tricuspid Valve Replacement for Treating Severe Tricuspid Regurgitation. JACC Cardiovasc Interv [Internet]. 2020 Nov 9 [cited 2020 Dec 11];13(21):2482-93. Available from: https://linkinghub.elsevier.com/retrieve/pii/S1936879820314989

[55] Lu F, Qiao F, Lv Y, An Z, Liu X, Cao P, et al. A radial force-independent bioprosthesis for transcatheter tricuspid valve implantation in a preclinical model. Int J Cardiol [Internet]. 2020 Nov 15 [cited 2020 Dec 11];319:120-6. Available from: http://www.internationaljournalofcardiology.com/article/S0167527320334483/fulltext

[56] F. L, Z. X, X. M, H. Z, F. Q, Z. S, et al. TCT-94 A Radial Force-Independent Bioprosthesis for Transcatheter Tricuspid Valve Implantation:

First-in-Man Clinical Trial. J Am Coll Cardiol. 2019;

[57] TRISCEND Study.

[58] Kolte D, Elmariah S. Transcatheter Tricuspid Valve Therapy. Curr Treat Options Cardiovasc Med [Internet]. 2019 Jun 18 [cited 2020 Dec 11];21(6):26. Available from: http://link.springer.com/10.1007/s11936-019-0730-7

[59] Laule M, Stangl V, Sanad W, Lembcke A, Baumann G, Stangl K. Percutaneous transfemoral management of severe secondary tricuspid regurgitation with edwards sapien XT bioprosthesis: First-in-man experience [Internet]. Vol. 61, Journal of the American College of Cardiology. J Am Coll Cardiol; 2013 [cited 2020 Dec 11]. p. 1929-31. Available from: https://pubmed.ncbi.nlm.nih.gov/23500268/

[60] Dreger H, Mattig I, Hewing B, Knebel F, Lauten A, Lembcke A, et al. Treatment of Severe TRIcuspid regurgitation in patients with advanced heart failure with caval vein implantation of the edwards sapien XT valve (TRICAVAL): A randomised controlled trial. EuroIntervention [Internet]. 2020 Apr 1 [cited 2020 Dec 11];15(17):1506-13. Available from: https://pubmed.ncbi.nlm.nih.gov/31929100/

[61] Mattig I, Knebel F, Hewing B, Stangl V, Stangl K, Laule M, et al. Impact of inferior caval valve implantation on severity of tricuspid regurgitation and right heart function. Echocardiography [Internet]. 2020 Jul 14 [cited 2020 Dec 11];37(7):999-1007. Available from: https://onlinelibrary.wiley.com/doi/abs/10.1111/echo.14760

[62] Lauten A, Figulla HR, Unbehaun A, Fam N, Schofer J, Doenst T, et al. Interventional Treatment of Severe Tricuspid Regurgitation. Circ Cardiovasc Interv [Internet]. 2018 Feb 1 [cited 2020 Dec 11];11(2). Available from: https://pubmed.ncbi.nlm.nih.gov/29445001/

[63] Lauten A, Ferrari M, Hekmat K, Pfeifer R, Dannberg G, Ragoschke-Schumm A, et al. Heterotopic transcatheter tricuspid valve implantation: First-in-man application of a novel approach to tricuspid regurgitation. Eur Heart J [Internet]. 2011 May [cited 2020 Dec 11];32(10):1207-13. Available from: https://pubmed.ncbi.nlm.nih.gov/21300731/

[64] Toggweiler S, De Boeck B, Brinkert M, Buhmann R, Bossard M, Kobza R, et al. First-in-man implantation of the Tricento transcatheter heart valve for the treatment of severe tricuspid regurgitation. EuroIntervention [Internet]. 2018 Sep 1 [cited 2020 Dec 11];14(7):758-61. Available from: https://pubmed.ncbi.nlm.nih.gov/29969434/

[65] Montorfano M, Beneduce A, Ancona MB, Ancona F, Sgura F, Romano V, et al. Tricento Transcatheter Heart Valve for Severe Tricuspid Regurgitation: Procedural Planning and Technical Aspects. JACC Cardiovasc Interv [Internet]. 2019 Nov 11 [cited 2020 Dec 11];12(21):e189-91. Available from: https://linkinghub.elsevier.com/retrieve/pii/S1936879819315213

[66] Werner P, Russo M, Scherzer S, Aref T, Coti I, Mascherbauer J, et al. Transcatheter Caval Valve Implantation of the Tricento Valve for Tricuspid Regurgitation Using Advanced Intraprocedural Imaging. JACC Case Reports [Internet]. 2019 Dec [cited 2020 Dec 11];1(5):720-4. Available from: https://linkinghub.elsevier.com/retrieve/pii/S2666084919304735

[67] Orban M, Rommel KP, Ho EC, Unterhuber M, Pozzoli A, Connelly KA, et al. Transcatheter Edge-to-Edge Tricuspid Repair for Severe Tricuspid Regurgitation Reduces Hospitalizations

for Heart Failure. JACC Hear Fail. 2020 Apr 1;8(4):265-76.

[68] Taramasso M, Alessandrini H, Latib A, Asami M, Attinger-Toller A, Biasco L, et al. Outcomes After Current Transcatheter Tricuspid Valve Intervention: Mid-Term Results From the International TriValve Registry. JACC Cardiovasc Interv [Internet]. 2019 Jan 28 [cited 2020 Dec 11];12(2):155-65. Available from: https://pubmed.ncbi.nlm.nih.gov/30594510/

[69] Taramasso M, Benfari G, van der Bijl P, Alessandrini H, Attinger-Toller A, Biasco L, et al. Transcatheter Versus Medical Treatment of Patients With Symptomatic Severe Tricuspid Regurgitation. J Am Coll Cardiol [Internet]. 2019 Dec 17 [cited 2020 Dec 11];74(24):2998-3008. Available from: https://pubmed.ncbi.nlm.nih.gov/31568868/

[70] Lurz P, Orban M, Besler C, Braun D, Schlotter F, Noack T, et al. Clinical characteristics, diagnosis, and risk stratification of pulmonary hypertension in severe tricuspid regurgitation and implications for transcatheter tricuspid valve repair. Eur Heart J [Internet]. 2020 Aug 1 [cited 2020 Dec 11];41(29):2785-95. Available from: https://pubmed.ncbi.nlm.nih.gov/32176280/

[71] Stocker TJ, Hertell H, Orban M, Braun D, Rommel K-P, Ruf T, et al. Cardiopulmonary Hemodynamic Profile Predicts Mortality After Transcatheter Tricuspid Valve Repair in Chronic Heart Failure. JACC Cardiovasc Interv [Internet]. 2020 Dec [cited 2020 Dec 11]; Available from: https://linkinghub.elsevier.com/retrieve/pii/S1936879820319713

[72] D'Alto M, Naeije R. Transcatheter tricuspid valve repair in patients with pulmonary hypertension [Internet]. Vol. 41, European Heart Journal. Oxford University Press; 2020 [cited 2020 Dec 11]. p. 2811-2. Available from: https://academic.oup.com/eurheartj/article/41/29/2811/5865473

[73] Besler C, Unterhuber M, Rommel KP, Unger E, Hartung P, von Roeder M, et al. Nutritional status in tricuspid regurgitation: implications of transcatheter repair. Eur J Heart Fail [Internet]. 2020 Oct 26 [cited 2020 Dec 11];22(10):1826-36. Available from: https://onlinelibrary.wiley.com/doi/10.1002/ejhf.1752